Breastfeeding in Ramadan

A Guide for Fasting Mothers

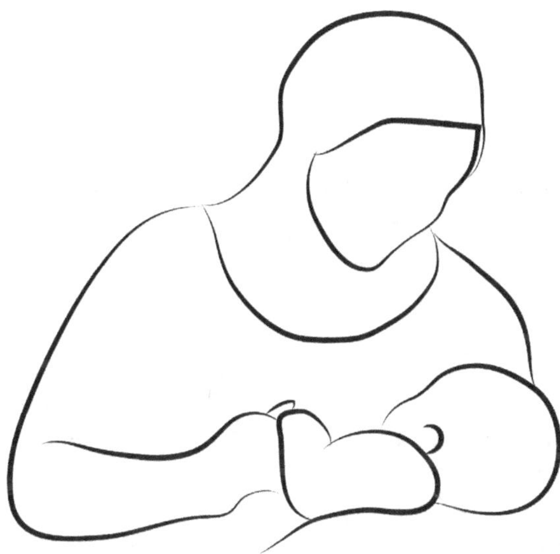

by Latonia Anthony

Printed in the United States of America

Ihya Press Publishing

Villa Park, IL

This book is not intended as a substitute for the medical advice of physicians. The reader should regularly consult a physician in matters relating to his/her health and particularly with respect to any symptoms that may require diagnosis or medical attention.

This book is not a substitute for the advice or information of a qualified Islamic scholar. Matters of fiqh, shariah law, aqeedah and tafsir should be addressed to the appropriate individuals in your community or abroad.

This book is not a substitute for seeing a lactation consultant.

Contents

Chapter 1

A Mother's Fast

Introduction

In the Name of Allah, Most Gracious, Ever Merciful.

Breastmilk is a superfood. By Allah's infinite wisdom it has several benefits and is the best nutrition in the first two years of life. Children have a right to milk and mothers gain reward for honoring the bond of nursing. The goal of this book is to help the many sisters whom take on the challenge of fasting while breastfeeding. Any good in it is from Allah and any mistakes are from me, May Allah forgive me.

Mothers may breastfeed their children two complete years for whoever wishes to complete the nursing [period]. Upon the father is the mothers' provision and their clothing according to what is acceptable. No person is charged with more than his capacity. No mother should be harmed through her child, and no father through his child. And upon the [father's] heir is [a duty] like that [of the father]. And if they both desire weaning through mutual consent from both of them and consultation, there is no blame upon either of them. And if you wish to have your children nursed by a substitute, there is no blame upon you as long as you give payment according to what is acceptable. And fear Allah and know that Allah is Seeing of what you do. (Surah Al Baqarah, Verse 233)

Many people are at odds about nursing mothers fasting. It seems like a conflict, not eating and making milk. Rather it is a balancing act. One that is amazingly possible with the right preparation. The intermittent Muslim fast is quite safe compared to other non-Muslim fasts that involve not eating for 24 hours or more. This dawn to dusk fast varies in length and gets shorter as the month passes. For the healthy well-nourished woman this allows enough time to eat and drink. With proper rest and monitoring, it is possible to fast without damaging the breastfeeding relationship. For many the risks outweigh the benefits, to become spiritually rejuvenated and bond with family in this special time of year. There is a permissible exemption during Ramadan for mothers who have a fear for themselves or their child. The fasts should be made-up (qadha) at a later time. Preferably, before the next Ramadan.

And We have enjoined upon man care for his parents. His mother carried him, increasing her in weakness upon weakness, and his weaning is in two years. Be grateful to Me and to your parents; to Me is the final destination (Surah Luqman, Verse 14)

Benefits of Breastfeeding

- Natural, wholesome food

- Prevents allergies, asthma and diabetes

- low risk of obesity

- Protects from diseases

- Easily digests

- Reduces SIDS

- Higher IQ

- Better dental health

- More bonding

- Breastmilk is always free and ready

Breastfeeding also prevents cancer, osteoporosis, hemorrhage, and depression for mothers.

It is a myth that fasting in an Islamic manner causes low milk supply. Unfortunately this message has pervaded some Muslim communities so much that mothers don't care to discuss fasting or take an effort to be evaluated to determine if they can. Studies on West African Muslimahs (whom often fast while breastfeeding), show that fasting does not cause low milk supply. But it can change the composition a little. Breastmilk is always changing so this is not detrimental. In fact depending on the time of day, the age of a child and mother's diet, breastmilk is a custom blend with each feed, Allahu Akbar! Plus the fast is temporary, lasting no more than 30 days in Ramadan. Once the fast has ended and mother begins eating and drinking throughout the day, the milk returns to her typical pattern of production. However, mothers must be warned. Breastmilk will diminish from dehydration. Hydrating overnight and resting will prevent this. A nation suffering from famine or drought can also lead to low milk supply for obvious reasons.

> *Your wealth and your children are but a trial, and Allah has with Him a great reward. (Surah Taghabun 64, verse 15)*

It is my firm belief that if we trust in Allah (swt) and make intention to gain His pleasure by fasting, He will provide all the sustenance needed for the baby and mother. From my personal experience, I have noticed an increase in my milk when I put more trust in Allah and worried less about missing lunch. By His mercy, he has given the breastfeeding mother an allowance to abstain from fasting should a fear arise for her child or herself.

Should I Fast?

If you have a genuine fear that breastfeeding and fasting will harm you or your child you can make-up your fasts later. Allah is most Merciful, and there are many ways to participate in Ramadan and other holidays (see last section). If you choose to forego fasting ensure your excuse is valid by means of advice from a reliable Muslim opinion, previous experience or clear, unmistakable signs.

> *The month of Ramadhan is that in which was revealed the Qur'an, a guidance for the people and clear proofs of guidance and criterion. So whoever sights the new moon of the month, let him fast it; and whoever is ill or on a journey - then an equal number of other days. Allah intends for you ease and does not intend for you hardship and [wants] for you to complete the period and to glorify Allah for that [to] which He has guided you; and perhaps you will be grateful. (Surah al Baqarah, verse 185)*

The Prophet (peace and blessings of Allaah be upon him) said: "Allah has relieved the traveller of the obligation of fasting and half of the prayer, and He has relieved the pregnant woman and nursing mother of the obligation of fasting." al-Tirmidhi, 715; Ibn Maajah, 1667

Women who have a baby less than six months old (whom make almost 1 liter of breastmilk a day), live in hot climates, are low income, tandem nurse, have multiples e.g. twins and who are older than 35 years are most at risk of severe dehydration and should not fast until weaning has occurred. The same goes for women who have confirmed low milk supply, must supplement, have a child that is underweight (preemies) or ill, take medications or have health conditions that make it difficult to breastfeed. If a mother really wants to fast, she can do partial fasting- committing to two to three days a week.

Mission Impossible

Fasting affects each woman and her nursling differently. One mother may struggle to keep up her supply, while another does fine. High-risk women who are nursing an infant less than 6 months and live in hot climates obviously should be advised not to fast. But many able-bodied moms with older babies and toddlers fast successfully. I can remember the glaring eyes and hostile responses when I was nursing my second daughter, "But sister, why?! You are exempt from fasting." I appreciated their concern for me but we must be careful with our deen. Breastfeeding is not a free pass from fasting in Ramadan, contrary to popular belief. Nor is it a token to be used as an excuse to be laidback in our worship. The reformation during Ramadan make us healthier spiritually and physically. This special opportunity to boost faith and worship is not easy to pass up, even when it's hard to fast.

Also, mothers should consider that making up accumulated days of fasting can be difficult. Especially if you get pregnant again before they are made-up. Mother's of stair-step children understand this best. Breastfeeding while fasting has risks but is possible. Breastfeeding is still a mystery to many who do not know that our bodies are amazing and will preserve the milk supply even in extreme conditions such as in malnourished women who barely get one meal a day. And we all know how much food we eat at meals during Ramadan is more than enough for one day! Fasting is definitely not for every woman, but it is possible when done with proper care.

Fasting is something done in private, between the individual and Allah. As I always tell women, "Only you know your body and it's limitations. Make the decision that is right for you. If you choose not to fast, there are other ways to participate during Ramadan. However, if you do fast you must be aware of your body's needs." Warning signs include constipation, dark urine, vomiting, dizziness, fatigue and headache. Any combination of these symptoms is your body telling you that it is not getting enough fluids. If you experience these, assess your situation and seek medical attention. If you suspect your health is in trouble aside from the ordinary discomforts of fasting (detoxing), it is permissible to break your fast and make it up another day. A day or two of rest will help replenish your body. Go with your instinct and stop fasting if necessary. Allah is Merciful and would not want you to hurt yourself when he has given you an excuse to delay fasting. It is also beneficial to be aware of the strength of your let down and your baby's state e.g. are they more agitated or less playful. Do not ignore warning signs that could compromise your breastfeeding relationship or your health.

Fasting Checklist

1. My nifas (postpartum bleeding) has ended and I am not currently menstruating

2. I am in good health. I do not have any illnesses or take medications that would make fasting dangerous

3. My child's growth and development is normal

4. I have made preparations to help manage my household so I can get proper rest

5. Any issues with breastfeeding e.g. nipple pain, or poor latch, have been properly addressed and treated to the best of my ability

6. My milk supply sustains my child. If not, I comfortably use a milk substitute or solid foods to supplement my child.

7. I am committed to focusing on hydrating and eating right during Ramadan

8. If married, my husband supports my decision to fast

9. I understand that there is a risk of my milk supply lowering and that breastfeeding challenges can arise while fasting

10. I am aware of warning signs of dehydration. I will seek medical attention if necessary

11. I know how to contact a lactation consultant for help

12. I have a support network of friends or family

13. I have made intention to fast, fisabilillah

Chapter 2

Barriers to Breastfeeding

There are many practices that keep mothers from successfully fasting and maintaining their milk supply in Ramadan.

1. Formula: A study by Ertem showed that 23% of mothers give supplements during Ramadan. Supplementing with artificial milk causes mothers to skip feedings. The breast is not emptied, the brain does not get a cue that a baby needs to be fed and the body slows milk production. Introducing formula to replace breastfeeding, especially during Ramadan will lower milk supply. Formula also takes longer to digest so a child may not wake up as often to eat. If needed, supplementing with 1-2 small cups of breastmilk is better. If your supply drops significantly stop fasting. Also note that introducing formula to a breastfed baby changes their healthy gut lining and may trigger stomach issues and allergies.

2. Bottles: Introducing even one bottle can be a slippery slope. If the child is less than a year, they may get nipple confusion or start refusing the breast. Babies often favor bottles because the flow is fast and it requires little energy on their part. If you must bottlefeed, choose one that mimics the breast and use it sparingly. For example, once mid-afternoon. An exclusively breastfed baby will drink from a cup or spoon much better than

a bottle. Also, caregivers have more control to pace feedings so the child is not gulping down their milk. Letting a baby drink too fast can cause them to become very fussy at the breast where they must suckle to stimulate a letdown.

3. Schedules: Feeding schedules are not natural or nurturing. A child less than two years should not be told they cannot eat. Feeding them in a timely manner establishes trust and maintains the milk supply. Watch your baby not the clock.

4. Night weaning: Babies consume 20% of their milk at night. The body makes the most milk at night because prolactin levels are highest at this time, particularly from 2am-6am. Prolactin regulates the milk supply and rises from suckling so it is very beneficial to nurse at night. Night are busy during Ramadan but nursing mothers must take it easy. Rest, hydration and feeding the baby are priority. If you feel lonely because everyone else is at the mosque, organize a mother's night of prayer with lots of snacks, water, pillows and helpers for the children. Even one night will be tremendously rewarding.

5. Complete weaning: In some places women are advised to stop breastfeeding to fast Ramadan. This is unnecessary and takes away the child's right to optimal nutrition, breastmilk. Each woman should assess her situation individually and should not feel like she has to stop breastfeeding. If there is substantial fear the woman should not fast at all, it can be made up later.

6. Birth Control: Estrogen containing contraceptives like combo pills or the patch cause milk supply to lower. If you must use hormones, choose a progesterone only pill. Barrier methods like the diaphragm or charting are safer.

7. Homebound Nursing: It's easily said but not always done to nurse in public. As Muslimahs we are modest and must protect our awrah but a mother has to feed her child too. Islam approves nursing outside your home for this reason. It's best to

be practical and relax- women have breastfed their children for thousands of years and it was not a special event. Breastmilk is readily available, warm and clean. It was meant to be portable and convenient for families. So find a comfortable spot, and let your baby eat. Use a nursing cover, goto your car, or use a quiet room if one is available. If you attend any extended events or trips, bring a breast pump if you will be separated from your child. You should pump just as often as your child eats. This prevents clogged ducts and keeps your supply up.

8. Negativity: Share your decision to fast with close family and friends. But avoid people who will stress you out. Anxiety and worry can make it longer for you to have a letdown. Overtime stress causes low milk supply.

Breastmilk is Resilient

Even when women are not fasting, they commonly think they do not make enough milk. My sisters, we worry too much. Studies have shown that short term fasting does not lower milk supply, which is commonly caused from poor latching, infrequent feeds, and sucking problems. In one study 22% of mothers who thought that their milk was lower showed no signs of low milk supply. In a UAE study, milk samples were taken from healthy mothers before and after Ramadan. It found that fasting did not negatively effect breastmilk. Macronutrients such as proteins and carbohydrates stayed the same. Fat had little or no change. The breasts make some milk fats. So, if it is not in the mother's diet it will be taken from her body. Micronutrients such as potassium, magnesium and zinc did alter. Yet, these are only needed in small amounts and milk is constantly changing to meets baby's needs. Therefore, this temporary change was not significant. Plus mother's diet and taking a multivitamin can prevent these changes.

A study by Rakicioglu et al 2006 looked at 2-5 month old infants during Ramadan and found that fasting had no effect on baby's weight. They did note that if a mother did not drink adequate fluids the baby would breastfeed as usual that day and feed more frequently the following two days. It is recommended to increase fluid intake starting two days before a fast. Lastly, some studies found that mothers ate more carbs and fat and gained up to 1kg during Ramadan despite eating less than the dietary recommendations. Studies have also shown that in mothers who lose weight due to fasting, milk remained the same. In conclusion breastmilk quality and composition is generally unaffected by Ramadan fasting.

Blood Sugar and Breastmilk

When you eat your body converts food to energy. The extra energy is stored as glycogen in the liver, muscles or fat cells. Whenever the body needs some spare energy it takes it from these resources. However the brain, nervous system and blood cells primarily use glucose from the bloodstream. Not glycogen, like the rest of the body. Lactocytes, the milk-making cells in the breast also need glucose in order to make lactose. Lactose is the main sugar in breastmilk, providing 40% of the calories. It decreases the unhealthy bacteria in baby's tummy, helping improve the absorption of important minerals, such as magnesium, calcium, and phosphate. For this reason, it is crucial that lactating women eat suhoor and get proper nutrients at night to refuel their body.

If a woman is malnourished and has used all of her body's stores, it will breakdown scraps of fat molecules into ketone bodies and take muscle for protein. If a person is starving and the body begins to depend on this back-up process, it can be very dangerous. Ordinarily, this should not happen to a healthy, fasting Muslim because there is ample time between iftar and suhoor to eat. The body usually comfortably adapts to the change in mealtimes after a few days. And people tend to gain weight as opposed to losing weight while fasting.

Yet again, it is important to eat right and listen to your body. You must take care of yourself in order to take care of your child.

Chapter 3

Key Tips

Indeed, it is Allah who is the continual Provider, the firm possessor of strength. (Surah Adh-Dhuriyat, Verse 58)

Many women from different religions including Hindus, Jews, and Christians, fast while breastfeeding. Studies have shown that short term fasting does not hinder milk production. The body naturally adapts to the lower caloric intake and maintains milk supply. Depending on your child's age, the climate, your diet and eating habits you may feel more drained than others during a fast. Also some women's breasts are more sensitive. So maintaining a good supply can be issue well before they start fasting. If you choose to fast, it is very important to hydrate, eat nutritiously dense foods and rest. Breastfeed as normal. Be patient, your child will need to adjust to new breastmilk and routine changes. Also, you will experience some detox symptoms such as a headache, cramping and irritability which can make fasting a true jihad.

If you are exclusively breastfeeding, you are most at risk of developing dehydration and must be conscious of your eating and drinking habits. Women who have a baby less than six months old (whom make almost 1 liter of breastmilk a day), live in hot climates, are low income, tandem nurse, have multiples e.g. twins and who are older than 35 years are most at risk of severe dehydration and should not fast until weaning has occured. The same goes for women who have been diagnosed with low milk supply, have a child that is underweight (preemies) or ill, take medications or have health conditions that make it difficult to breastfeed.

Always consult with your doctor before taking on fasting while breastfeeding. Fasts can be easily made up after your child weans.

Staying Hydrated

Our bodies are mostly water. Breastmilk is 87% water. "Have those who disbelieved not considered that the heavens and the earth were a joined entity, and We separated them and made from water every living thing? Then will they not believe?" Surah Al Anbya verse 30. Despite it's importance, studies show that up to 75% of Americans do not drink enough water. They are chronically dehydrated. In Ramadan, we all experience mild dehydration when we are fasting. The body continuously loses fluids through sweating, breathing, urination. Lactating women have an extra demand on their bodies that contributes to dehydration. Therefore, it is very important do things that help conserve your body fluids until maghrib time when thirst is quenched, veins are moistened and the reward is confirmed, if Allah wills.

- Do indoor activities like crafting, board games, extra worship, memorization and community service. Cut off the television and enjoy your family.

- Infuse waters and make fresh juices like hibiscus and tamarind

- Take a cool, relaxing bath. Be careful not to swallow or inhale water

- Keep a water bottle and snack on you at all times even while you are fasting. You want to be prepared in case of an urgent situation in which you must stop fasting for the sake of you or your child's health.

- Wake up to drink water at least twice in the middle of the night. Aim for at least two liters from Maghrib to suhoor time. However avoid over drinking as too much water is harmful. To remind yourself to drink more often mark a large water bottle with a permanent marker. Draw a line for each hour, write the time and stick to this schedule. Even when you are sleepy, you must drink.

- Wear light colored, thin clothing made of natural fibers like cotton or linen

- Avoid lifting heavy objects

- Limit caffeine, high sugar drinks and dairy products. These include soda, coffee and tea.

- Eat high water content foods like watermelon, cucumber, and strawberries. Cook soups and broths. Twenty percent of fluids come from food.

- Exercise a few hours after iftar e.g. walking or light aerobics. This can help you to feel better and release toxins. Light stretching during the day also has benefits.

- Get proper rest. Nap 1-2 times a day. Pray tarawih at home instead of going out late at night.

- Sip water slowly

- Breastfeed in side lying or laidback position, with lots of pillows to allow your body to relax

- Avoid consuming too much acid forming, processed foods with refined sugars a.k.a. Junk Food.

- Eat little meat. It's a sunnah and it's best for your physical and spiritual health.

- Eat parsley, mint and sage in moderation. These herbs can dry up your milk! This includes mint tea, tabbouleh and sage tea (maramia).

- Have your medications reviewed by a lactation consultant

- Bond with your child. The hormones responsible for making milk are higher when you are close. Sleep near your child, baby-wear and do skin to skin contact. You will feel more relaxed and your milk will flow as the love hormone oxytocin rises. So snuggle and cuddle as much as you like. A ring sling or woven baby wrap worn on the back will allow you to move around and pray easily. Make your own by simply buying 4 to 6 yards of osnaburg/gauze fabric that is at least 30 inches wide. If want to be fancy you can hem it all around the edges. Learn to wrap your child on your back at www.thebabywearer.com.

Kick Bad Habits...

Many women go about Ramadan overeating at iftar (meal to break fast at sunset), drinking caffeinated beverages such as soda and black tea, indulging on sweets, staying awake all night or habitually skipping suhoor (morning meal before fast). They also spend the day shopping, cooking, cleaning, taking care of children and preparing for guests. Then they wonder why they have a horrible headache by noon. Though Ramadan is a time we enjoy more gatherings and celebrate with rich meals, it is not what this holy month is truly about. While the Shaytan is locked up and the doors of mercy are open there are so many spiritual benefits for us to take advantage of during this short period.

Fasting should be an act we do with pure intentions, and which should bring reflection and tranquility to our hearts. It is a time to strengthen our iman (faith) while our bodies are weak. It is only during this time that we realize how distracting the desire to eat is and how dependent we are on Allah for our sustenance. If you are breastfeeding and fasting, listen to your body- sit down and rest if you feel tired, eat suhoor so your brain has energy during the day, eat normal servings, and focus on hydrating your body with plenty of pure water. Remember, everyone experiences physical challenges while fasting that they must overcome. However, fasting can be very invigorating and spiritually uplifting once we realize it!

Keep Your Cool

Fasting is known to make people feel more irritable and drowsy during the day. Therefore it's no surprise that mother's must work harder to "keep their cool." Let's face it, most of us experience sleep deprivation and stress everyday. A mother's work is never done. Fasting truly exercises our patience. It is important to be calm and have self-control in order to care for your family without getting burned out. Safety is another concern because more accidents occur in this distracting state. Ramadan truly tests us whether we are fasting or not, changing our routines and circadian rhythms. You may be preparing larger meals or staying up at night. Plus taking care of an infant or busy toddler. In times of high tension, take a deep breath. Remove yourself from the situation. It is not worth it to spend your energy on becoming upset. Anger itself can disturb your fast. So if it occurs, lower yourself by sitting or laying. Be quiet instead of yelling, backbiting or swearing. Make wudu. Seek refuge with Allah from Shaytan. If you become agitated with your baby put them in safe place, like a crib and call someone to takeover. Take deep breaths and count to ten. It may help to take the child for a walk in the stroller, car ride, bath, or give them a pacifier.

Who spend in the cause of Allah during ease and hardship and who restrain anger and who pardon the people - and Allah loves the doers of good. (Surah al Imran, Verse 134)

Stay Focused

It easy to get caught up with caring for children and hunger pangs. Yet, Ramadan is a time of devotion to Allah. Renew your intentions often and keep company with individuals that strengthen your iman. Ask Allah for forgiveness and repent. Remind yourself of the ultimate goal of fasting and the tremendous mercy in the month of Ramadan. Carry a mini-book of Quran or duas like Fortress of a Muslim to read in your down time. You could also download these onto a smart device. Listen to seerah or lectures when you are busy cooking or caring for children.

Expect an Adjustment period

It will take anywhere from 3 to 14 days for your body and your baby to get used to the new routine. You may experience softer breasts during the day, more frequent nursing sessions at night and a fussier child occasionally. These are normal expectations of fasting while breastfeeding and do not necessarily indicate true low milk supply. An infant or toddler may not understand why their daytime feeds suddenly flow slower. So make sure you spend more time playing and bonding with them.

Know When to Stop

You heard it right sisters. If you are having real issues with breast-feeding your child you need to take a break from fasting. Feeding them takes priority and these days can be made up at a later time. Meet with a lactation consultant for help to resolve any issues or advice on how to supplement.

Chapter 4

Father's Role

In these modern times it is common for Muslim women to feel isolated as converts, new moms, or homemakers. Be by your wife's side to guide and comfort her. Successful nursing requires time, patience and much energy from mothers.

Fathers have a unique and important role when it comes to breastfeeding, too. Ultimately, they are responsible for ensuring the child is properly fed because it considered a part of their maintenance. This means he supports his wife and appreciates that she is providing the healthiest milk to their child. But, fathers cannot force women to breastfeed. Alternatives include hiring a wet-nurse, buying expressed milk from another woman, or purchasing formula. If he cannot afford these options or the child won't take another woman's milk, the mother should breastfeed if she is capable of it.

A father's work of providing for the family, balances duties and ensures everyone's basic needs are met. In a hadith narrated in Sahih Bukhari and Sahih Muslim, The Prophet (pbuh), was reported to have said: "Each of you is a shepherd and each of you is responsible for his flock. The leader is a shepherd of his people and is responsible for his flock; a man is the shepherd of his family and is responsible for his flock; a woman is the shepherd in the house of her husband and is responsible for her flock; a servant is the shepherd of his master's wealth and is responsible for it. Each of you is a shepherd and is responsible for his flock." Fathers play an important role in breast-feeding, the most obvious being providing for the family.

The financial support of fathers is an excellent duty which should not be disregarded. As translated narration of Thauban bin Bujdud (ra) states, The Prophet (saws) said: "The most excellent dinar is one a person spends on his family" (Imam Al-Nawawi's Riyad-us-Saliheen, Chapter 36 Sustentation of the Members of the Family).

If your child's mother wants to try fasting and there are no concerns, support her efforts. But sometimes no matter how strong a mother feels, fasting is not the best option. If this is the case, kindly express your concerns and tell her that she should delay fasting. If you both disagree talk about it with a counselor or help her make a plan to make the fast up when the child is older. Volunteer to fast with her on these days. Regardless, encourage her to increase her acts of ibadah and form better habits. Buy your wife healthy foods (she may need a cookbook for ideas) and help her around the house. For example, you can help chop vegetables or do a load of laundry.

Nursing moms need rest and fluids. Do not allow her to serve others without breaking her fast first, eating a small meal, drinking a bottle of water and nursing the baby.

Aisha – May Allah be pleased with her – was asked about the manners of the Prophet in his home? She replied: He was helping in doing the family duties and when he hears the call of prayer he goes out. Narrated by: Aisha – Degree: Right – the narrator: Al-Bukhari – The Source: Al-Jame' Al-Sahih – Page or number: 5363

If she needs a new khimar, vitamins or a baby wrap, find a way to get her these items. Allow her to rest and take the baby for a walk or with you to the mosque for prayer. Make sure she is not too stressed or experiencing depression. Limit visitors and gatherings at the home if possible. Allow her to attend halaqas outside the home or community iftars. If you both decide to start weaning, helpout with this transition which can be very stressful for her especially at night. Let her know that you appreciate her.

Lastly keep in mind the following hadith recorded by Muslim, the Prophet Muhammad (pbuh), was reported to have said (translation): "This world is all temporary conveniences, and the greatest joy in this life is a righteous wife."

Chapter 5

Preparing for Ramadan

Allah is the source of all sustenance. Let Him know your intentions. Ask him to fill your breasts with milk and give you a good supply while fasting. Remember the miracle of how Halima Sayida's (as) bosom suddenly filled, flowing with milk when she nursed the Prophet (pbuh) for the first time. Her baby had cried all night in hunger due to them not having anything to eat. However once she became Muhammed's (pbuh) wet-nurse, she had enough milk for both of them. Even her malnourished animals gave milk that provided an abundance of blessing for her family. Whenever thirst strikes (which is normal), make dua. If fear arises say "Audhu billahi mina shaytan ir-ajim" or "I seek refuge in Allah from the accursed Satan."

Think of the thirst Baraqah, the one our Nabi (pbuh) called "Ya Umm" or "O Mother" experienced when she made hijrah alone on foot while fasting. Allah provided a bucket a water for her out of nowhere and kept her from experiencing thirst for the rest of her life.

Every morning and evening say: "Allah is sufficient for me. There is no God but He. I have placed my trust in Him, He is Lord of the Majestic Throne." Whoever says this seven times in the morning after fajr, and seven times after Asr, Allah will take care of whatever worries him of the matter of this world and the hereafter.

The Prophet is reported to have said said: "Whoever says (when he leaves his house) – Bismillaah, tawakkaltu 'alaa Allaah, wa laa hawla wa laa quwwata illaa billaah – In the name of Allah, I put my trust in Allah and there is no power and no strength except with Allah- , it will be said to him: You are taken care of and you are protected and guided, and the devils will move away from him, and one devil says: What can you do with a man who has been guided, taken care of and protected?" [Abu Dawood, At-Tirmidhi]

Try your best to stay in wudu or a state of spiritual purification. Pray for strength to make it through the day. Be thankful and think of other women who fast but have less than you. In some countries, mothers are fasting yet they have more children to care for and less food to prepare a meal with, SubhanAllah. Many of our sisters are spending Ramadan in war torn areas in constant fear of bombs and shootings, or they live in a refugee camp. Allah is Most Merciful. Find peace in knowing that he provides for us all each day.

Buy a Galactagogue

A galactagogue is a substance that increases milk supply. Giving yourself a boost before Ramadan will help prevent low milk supply as you transition to different eating patterns and fasting. Also if you decide to start pumping before Ramadan, it will help maintain your present supply. The most popular galactagogue is a herb called Fenugreek (hulbah in arabic) and can be taken as a liquid extract, dried powder capsule or in tea form. In many Arab cultures it is served as a sweet dish or drink to new mothers. It is a great supplement because it is safe and has a long history of use without serious side effects. Not only is Fenugreek super at increasing milk, it can also be gargled for a sore throat, used to stimulate appetite and aids in digestion. Also, all my breastfeeding moms will be happy to know that its seeds can be steeped, mashed and applied to the breasts to relieve mastitis and engorgement! It is reported that the Prophet Muhammed (pbuh) once said "If my people knew what was in fenugreek, they would have bought and paid it's weight in gold.

Fenugreek can be found at most Arab or Indian grocery stores because it is commonly used as spice in curry dishes. You can also cook stuffed rotis, paranthas, stews and vegetables with it. It is also as a supplement at health food stores but will be more expensive. Alternatively one may buy the seeds and make tea (known as methi ki chai in India). You can steep a few teaspoons in a pot of hot water and fill a pitcher to be kept in the refrigerator. Drink a cup 2-3 times day. Milk supply will significantly increase within 24-72 hours and you can stop using it once milk supply increases. If you are allergic to chickpeas or peanuts, do not take Fenugreek. Those with thyroid or blood sugar issues should avoid it as well. This may make you smell like maple syrup.

Smart Tips:

- Smart Tip #1: Take a pill that contains a complete postnatal vitamin and a supplement to increase milk supply. For example the Milkies Nursing Blend Breastfeeding Supplement, which contains vitamins, minerals and herbs. It is vegan and can be purchased from www.fairhavenhealth.com. This will save you money and time. Plus, you will not have to take an extra prenatal vitamin because it has everything in it. It is an all-in-one supplement.

- Smart Tip #2: The taste of fenugreek can be off putting or cause stomach discomfort. Put fresh, ground fenugreek into sweet treats such as cookies or muffins. To save yourself time consider purchasing fenugreek bars from Mrs. Patel at www.mrsmilk.com. Based on Indian Ayurveda, her bars have good reviews and she also sells tea.

Another option is to buy Motherlove's Alcohol-Free More Milk Plus Formula because it is convenient and is easy to take.

How to Make a Tincture

A strong, herbal extract will save you time and money. Fill a mason jar half way with a 1/4 to 1/2 cup each of several herbs such as fenugreek, fennel, nettle, goat's rue, and blessed thistle. These herbs are known to increase and enrich milk. Add enough hot water to moisten the herbs. Fill the jar a half inch from the top with vegetable glycerin. After closing the jar tightly, place it in a slow cooker with a small towel underneath to keep the jar from breaking. Fill the slow cooker with water up to the top of the jar (not touching the lid). Place lid on top, it probably will not close all the way. Leave it on the lowest setting for 3 days. The jar will be hot but not boiling. Add water as necessary. After 3 days, strain the herbal mixture through a cheesecloth into a glass container. Squeeze the herbs a bit, pour a small amount of boiling water over them, and throw them away. Close tightly and label the tincture. This will last 14-24 months. Take 2-3 droppers twice a day.

*If you do not own a slow cooker you can let the jar sit in a dark place for 6 weeks. Give it a shake each day.

Sudani Fenugreek Pudding Recipe (Madeedah Hilba)

Ingredients:

- 2 cans evaporated milk

- 4 tbsp sugar

- 1/4 cup Fenugreek seeds

- 1 Tbsp corn starch

- 1 Tbsp flour

- 1/4 cup cold milk

In a medium sauce pan, pour the 2 cans of evaporated milk, fenugreek and sugar and bring to a boil. While that is going, in a bowl dissolve the the flour and cornstarch in cold milk. Once the ingredients in the saucepan are starting to simmer, turn down the heat to medium low, then add the cold milk/flour/starch mix to the pan and keep mixing constantly with a whisk. You want to mix it frequently so it doesn't clump. It should develop the thick pudding consistency. You may need to add more milk/starch/flour to the mix if you are not getting it to be thick enough. This should take about 10-20 minutes.

Most Common Herbs and Foods Used to Increase Milk Supply

- Alfalfa (Medicago sativa) Dose: Up to 60 g daily (1 to 2 capsules 4 times a day) Other uses: Diuretic and laxative Caution: Alfalfa may cause loose stools and/or photosensitivity; do not use if allergic to peanuts and/or legumes; do not use in patients with systemic lupus erythematosus (SLE)

- Anise (Anisi fructus) Dose: 3.5 to 7 g as tincture or tea, 5 to 6 times a day Other uses: For anxiety and as antiflatulent Caution: Anise may cause allergic reaction

- Blessed Thistle (Cnici benedicti herba) Dose: Up to 2 g, in capsule form, daily Other uses: May increase appetite and settle upset stomach Caution: Blessed thistle may cause allergic reaction

- Borage (Borago officinalis) Dose: 1 to 2 g, in capsule form or as tincture, daily Other uses: For anxiety and as diuretic Caution: Borage may cause loose stools and/or minor gastrointestinal upset; avoid large amounts because of potential blood thinner action

- Caraway (Carvi fructus) Dose: 1.5 to 6 g daily as tincture, tea, or essential oil Other uses: For anxiety and as antiflatulent Caution: Avoid large amounts of the essential oil form (can be irritating to mucous membranes)

- Chaste Tree Fruit, Chasteberry,Vitex (Agni casti fructus) Dose: 30 to 40 mg daily as an extract Other uses: To treat breast pain dysmenorrhea Caution: Herb may cause rash

- Coriander, Cilantro (Coriandri fructus) Dose: 3 g daily as tea Other uses: Antiflatulent, diuretic, and mild antidiabetic Caution: Herb may rarely cause photo-sensitivity; avoid herb if allergic to celery; avoid large amounts of herb

- Dandelion (Taraxaci herba) Dose: 5 g, in capsule form or as tincture or tea, 3 times a day Other uses: Anti-diabetic and diuretic Caution: Dandelion may rarely cause contact dermatitis; patients with bile duct blockage, gall bladder problems, or bowel obstruction should not use

- Dill (Anethi fructus) Dose: 3 g daily as tincture or tea Other uses: Antiflatulent and diuretic Caution: None

- Fennel (Foeniculi fructus) Dose: 0.1 to 0.6 mL of oil (equal to 100 to 600 mg) daily Other uses: For gastrointestinal disorders and as an expectorant Caution: Fennel may cause allergic reaction and dermatitis

- Fenugreek (Foenugraeci semen) Dose: Orally, 6 g, in capsule form, daily; externally to treat inflammation, 50 g in 8 ounces of water Other uses: To stimulate appetite, externally to control inflammation Caution: Fenugreek may cause nausea and vomiting in mother and diarrhea in baby; may increase asthma symptoms or lower glucose levels in mother; may cause skin reactions with external use (avoid nipple area); may cause "maple syrup" smell in mother's and/or baby's urine and/or sweat; do not use if allergic to peanuts and/or legumes

- Garlic (Allii sativi bulbus) Dose: 4 to 9 g, in capsule form, daily Other uses: For possible positive cardio-vascular effects and/or immunesystem stimulation Caution: Garlic increases nursing time because of odor in breast milk but may decrease nursing time if garlic odor is unacceptable to infant

- Goat's Rue (Galegae officinalis herba) Dose: 1 to 2 mL of tincture, 2 to 3 times a day Other uses: To lower blood glucose levels Caution:None

- Hops (Lupuli strobulus) Dose: 500 mg of dry extract daily, 1 cup to 2 cups of tea daily, Other uses: For anxiety and insomnia Caution: None, but do not use hops if depressed

- Marshmallow Root (Althaeae radix) Dose: Two 500-mg capsules, in capsule form, 3 times a day; or 60g daily as tincture or tea Other uses: Diuretic Caution: Marshmallow root rarely may cause allergic reaction

- Milk Thistle (Cardui mariae herba) Dose: 12 to 15 g daily as infusion (equal to 200 to 400 mg of silibinin) Other uses: For possible liver protective properties Caution: Milk thistle may have laxative effect and/or cause allergic reaction

- Oat Straw, Oats (Avenaestramentum) Dose: 100 g daily Other uses: Diuretic and for anxiety and depression Caution: Do not use if patient has celiac disease

- Red Raspberry (Rubi idaei folium) Dose: 2.7 g as three 300-mg capsules 3 times a day or daily as tincture or tea Other uses: Nutritive Caution: Red raspberry rarely may cause loose stools and/or nausea; may decrease milk supply if used for greater than 2 weeks

- Red Clover (Trifolium pretense) Dose:40 to 80 mg daily as tincture or tea Other uses: For estrogenic properties and as expectorant Caution: Do not exceed recommended dosage; avoid fermented red clover; patients taking anticoagulants and/or aspirin should not use (contains coumarin, a blood thinner)

- Stinging Nettle (Urtica dioica and Urtica urens) Dose: 1.8 g as one 600-mg capsule 3 times a day, 1 cup of tea 2 to 3 times a day, 2.5 to 5.0 ml of tincture 3 times a day Other uses: Mild diuretic and for mild gastrointestinal upset Caution: Stinging

nettle may cause mild diuresis and/or mild gastrointestinal upset

- Vervain (Verbena officinalis) Dose: 30 to 50 g daily as tea Other
  uses: For anxiety and hypertension Caution: Do not use if pregnant (because of oxytocic properties)

Fast a Few Trial Days

Many people are challenged by the first few days of Ramadan. In addition to waking early for suhoor, unsatisfied hunger and thirst can be quite discomforting. Subhan' Allah, Allah is Merciful and provides us with so much barakah for fasting in the holy month. The transition from Shaban to fasting consistently in Ramadan can be eased if a few trial days are fasted before the start of Ramadan. This is especially true for a breastfeeding mother, who may experience more thirst and hunger than the average person. Prepare yourself by fasting one or two days a week and becoming familiar with how it will feel. This will also help prevent your milk supply from drastically changing or decreasing. If you fear dehydration, set a schedule to drink extra fluids during the night and see if it works for you. A breastfeeding woman needs 12-16 cups of fluid daily. Avoid caffeinated drinks such as soda, coffee and tea that can cause dehydration. Try different combinations and amounts of food to see what makes you most comfortable during the day. You may find that you are able to function with a lot less food despite breastmilk production burning about 200-500 calories a day. Depending on your activity level, you may need to consume more calories per day. However, these demands may change while fasting because the body's complex metabolic systems adapt to fasting, lowering caloric needs to maintain body function. For this reason, it is unnecessary to overeat at suhoor and iftar. Focus on quality of food and not quantity. Keep a simple food and fluid log to keep track of your progress and to develop a plan for Ramadan.

Most importantly, make dua that Allah (swt) gives you the strength to endure fasting despite the demands of your body while breastfeeding. Remember, it is not food alone that gives us the fuel to live in this world. Allah (swt), Ar-Razzaq (The Provider) is the ultimate source of all our physical and spiritual sustenance. Also, do not feel like this is a competition, if you have fear for the health of yourself, or your baby, it is permissible to make-up the fast at another time. May Allah (swt) make it easy for us all. Remember, It's not all or nothing Make intention to fast the whole of Ramadan but take things a day at a time. You may not be able to finish all 30 days. Or you may need to rest after 2 days. Remember, even one day of fasting in Ramadan has tremendous blessings. There is no reason to feel bad if it becomes too difficult. Allah is Most Merciful. Continue to pray and make daily devotions even if you aren't fasting.

Start Pumping

If you plan on breastfeeding during Ramadan this year, start pumping during Shaban (or earlier) and freeze the milk. Generally, twice a day evening and morning should be sufficient, but mothers of younger infants may be able to pump more often. This will provide a back-up supply, as your body adjusts to fasting. Many experience a temporary dip. Also if you are worried about your milk composition changing, this will ensure your baby gets all the nutrients he needs. Supplement with this breastmilk as much as you like and avoid using formula. This freezer stash will be your personal milk bank.

A breastfed baby will take expressed milk from a cup much easier than a bottle. Try the Doidy Cup or Medela's Softfeeder for a smaller baby. If the child does not take these well, try a spoon or dropper. It's best to avoid bottles and fake nipples. These can interfere with breastfeeding. You could also freeze it into popsicles or add it to baby cereal. If you wish, you can continue to pump at night during Ramadan to maintain your back-up supply for the future (or if your baby decides to have a growth spurt during Ramadan!). If you do not use the milk, it will be good for 3-6 months in the freezer.

Warm the milk by placing it in a bowl of warm water or holding it under running hot water. Do not boil or microwave breastmilk. Overheating destroys nutrients and could burn your child.

Gently swirl if cream sepearates.

Smart Tips:

1. Smart Tip: Your pumped milk may be wasted if your baby does not finish the bottles as expected. Prevent this from happening by storing small amount of milk separately. Freeze milk in ice cube trays and pop out into freezer bags each day. Label and store bags in the coldest part of the freezer.

2. Smart Tip: If you want to supplement your child with formula or expressed milk while keeping them at the breast, try a supplemental nursing system. A small tube will deliver extra milk when you are nursing.

Make a Chore Schedule

Take the burden off yourself and divide the housework (or hire a mommy's helper). Even small children can do chores like sweeping or putting clothes in the washer. If your family is not cooperative offer a reward or an allowance at the end of Ramadan. Let them know why it's important for them to help you. Children may like a task chart with stickers to mark off when their work is done. It gives them a sense of accomplishment. You could also write the chores on popsicle sticks and put them in jar. Have everyone pull one each day. This way it feels more like chance instead of them feeling like you are telling them to do something.

Plan Your Daily Devotions

Make a list of extra dhikr, prayers or Quran you want to read each day. Post it where you can see it or use a phone app to remind you to do them. You may want to schedule some days to do community service or help out at the masjid. This time management will help you reach your goals and gain more blessing inshAllah. If you need help making a list, download the free Daily Deeds Checklist as www.coachamal.com. Before Ramadan, it is also wise to write down people or things you want to make dua for each day.

Find another sister to be your Quran buddy. Together, you will motivate and encourage each other to read each day.

Clear Your Mind & Heart

Before and during Ramadan set aside time each day to reflect or meditate. Even 5 minutes a day will be beneficial to bring you peace of mind. Close your eyes and sit still. Try to focus and on a name of Allah or do tasbih. You can even do a particular salawat for the Prophet. It will also be helpful to journal. The Heart Wheel Journal created by Muhammed Al-Shareef is available free for download online. Take a walk outside and spend time with family to relax. You will be less stressed with these practices. It will also be easier to cope with daily challenges.

Smart Tip:

To ease stress use a calming spray. Mix 2 ounces of water with 20 drops of rosemary essential oil and 20 drops of lavender essential oil into a mister or spray bottle. Spray whenever you have a headache or when tension rises being careful not to get it in the nose or mouth. Chamomile essential oil is also great for relaxing, especially at bedtime.

Wake for Tahajjud

Before Ramadan, start waking up in the early hours and praying tahajjud. Suhoor will be roughly around the same time, before fajr. Grab a snack, make two rakats minimum, and nurse your child before jumping back into bed. This is a special time to repent and make dua, as they are more readily answered at this time. Ask Allah to bring you success this Ramadan and give you a good milk supply. This is also a quiet time to read your daily portion of Quran.

Prepare Meals in Advance

Buy in bulk. Do one weekly trip to the grocery store, with a prepared list.

Choose quality over quantity of food. Prepare and freeze one-pot dishes before Ramadan starts. Or you can do a few at the start of each week. Soups, curry, pizza and casseroles go well in the freezer. When you warm them for iftar make fresh bread, rice or salad to go with the meal. Freezing or refrigerating meat in marinade makes it flavorful and easy to prepare. Put it on the grill or roast it.

You can also make cooking easier by prepping foods in advance. The whole family can help chop vegetables. You can also use a food processor for this. Onions, garlic, and tomatoes are used often, so having these on hand will make meal prep quicker. Make broth and freeze it in an ice cube tray. Add 1-2 cubes to dishes to make it more flavorful.

You can also freeze or prepare homemade baby food. Use a small hand mill or blender and store it in an ice cube tray.

Another option is to prepare the evening meal in the morning. The meat can go in the slow cooker on low, which will allow it get juicy and tender. If you have multiple slow cookers you can do your sides and dessert in them as well. Using the slow cooker is also less mess and keeps the house cool.

Eat Slow

Take a pointer or two from the "Slow Food Movement". The Slow Food Movement began years ago to encourage people to stop eating unhealthy fast food. In the chaos of modern life, we have forgotten how to enjoy the simple things like a meal. With the exception of meat, all food comes from the Earth and has to grow slowly before it is harvested. Let's show our thanks by preparing and eating food in ways that is best for our physical and spiritual health.

1. It takes 20 minutes for the brain to realize you are full. Eating slower will make you eat less and essentially practice the sunnah of only filling a third of the stomach with food. It also promotes better digestion which starts in the mouth with careful chewing. You will be more mindful of what you are doing and enjoy the meal.

2. Eating slow also means eating with others like family, friend, and neighbors. There is more blessing and you will find there is plenty to share. Prepare a spread by putting a tablecloth on the floor with a few large dishes to share. Use your hands to eat instead of cutlery.

3. Eat slow-digesting carbs like yams, wild rice, and beans. These also include nuts, seeds, whole grains and vegetables (not starchy ones). These foods slowly increase blood glucose (low glycemic index) and cause a modest insulin release. They are high in fiber. They will give you energy slowly throughout the day. In contrast, refined sugar and processed foods like bagels, white rice, dinner rolls, rice cakes, cold cereal, and fat-free muffins hit the bloodstream quickly. They give a rush of energy and spike insulin. You are less likely to crash if you eat slow-digesting foods.

4. Eat local and seasonal produce as much as you can. Shop at the farmer's market or goto a nearby farm for your food. Fresh milk, eggs, herbs, vegetables and fruits have higher nutritional

content. They are also less likely to be genetically modified and have less pesticides. Some farmers also sell animals that you can hand slaughter (zabiha) and have processed on-site.

5. Eat homemade meals. These are most nutritious and whole-some. There is also more blessing in preparing family meals with loving hands, with wudu and remembrance of Allah.

Start Solids

If your child is older than 6 months it is good to start slowly in-troducing solids. This way your baby will be getting nutrients from both breastmilk and food. They may be able to go longer between breastfeeds because food digests slowly whereas breastmilk digest in about an hour. Don't force the child to eat if they don't want to. They may like it more if you mix your breastmilk in the food you give them. Use a hand mill or blender to quickly puree foods.

If your child is less than 6 months old, it is best give them only breastmilk.

Adjust Your Work Schedule

If you can take the whole month off, great. But many women have to work to support their family or serve their clients. Request a few days off in the beginning (when the fast is difficult) and near the end of the month. If possible reduce your hours each week or work half days. See if you can work from home or do your work online. Or request to start work earlier, in the evening or at night when it is cooler and you have more energy. If you prefer not to work and fast, work more hours in the 3 months before Ramadan and put the extra money in a savings. Take off for Ramadan and use this money for your expenses.

Plan Activities for Older Children

Keep your other children busy so you can take it easy. Stock up on supplies and do Ramadan theme crafts like Eid cards, paper lamps or a countdown calendar. Bake sugar cookies and have them decorate the house with garlands and posters. Go on outings like the children's museum, library or park to play. Choose places where you can sit and just supervise. Have them make goodie bags to hand out to other children at the mosque. Play board games as a family. Do mini halaqas to teach them about Islam.

Keep their hands busy with lacing cards, beading, or homemade play dough. For homeschooling, focus on workbooks or self-study. There are great Islamic workbooks at www.noorart.com for all ages. If you really need downtime let them watch educational movies or play games on a computer .

And do not feel guilty for this, mommies! If you don't have any, buy some Islamic DVDs like Zaky & Friends or Hooray for Baba Ali. Teach the children nasheeds or help them make up one with a tabla drum or hand clapping. Have them listen and memorize Quran. I use the 2 CD set Juz Amma Teacher with Children's Repetition by Mishary Rashid al-Afasy in the car and in my kid's bedroom. If neccesary to be afraid to seek help from a babysitter or family member to give you a much needed break at least once a week.

Chapter 6

During Ramadan

Abu Hurayra (Allah be pleased with him) said that the Prophet (Allah bless him & give him peace) said,
"The strong believer is better and more beloved to Allah than the weak believer, though there is good in both. Be avid for that which benefits you. Rely on Allah and do not deem yourself incapable..." [Muslim 4816, Ibn Majah 76, Ahmad 8436]

The month of Ramadan propels us into a better spiritual state. It drives us to be mindful of our intentions, practice and deeds. Parents often become burned out as they try to do everything like they did years before. Set realistic goals, Ramadan is not a marathon. Make sincere dua that the Almighty gives you sabr and strength, and that He helps you through this challenging time.

And Your Lord said: Call on Me, I will answer you Quran 40:60
Remember Me, and I will remember you, give thanks to Me, and reject Me not Quran 2:152

Remember, You are not alone

The female companions worried about their preoccupation with home and family duties. The men were always out with Rasullulah (pbuh), at the masjid, and learning about Allah (swt) and the hereafter.

Asmā' bint'l-Sakan al-Anṣāriyyah, on behalf of the women in Madīnah, approached the Prophet ṣallallāhu 'alayhi wa sallam (peace and blessings of Allāh be upon him) while surrounded by his companions. She boldly asked: "O Messenger of Allah! The men have taken all your time. . . " and she complained that men get the reward of the congregational prayers, Fridays, fighting with him and other works of good deeds while women were confined to their houses and taking care of their children. She asked if women get the same rewards. The Messenger of Allah ṣallallāhu 'alayhi wa sallam (peace and blessings of Allāh be upon him) replied, "Go back to the women who sent you and let them know that treating their husbands kindly and taking care of them is equivalent to that all you mentioned." Reported by al-Bazzar and al-Tabarāni

By nature women are nurturers. It is a blessing to be able to gain Allah's pleasure by simply caring for your family. Plus the reward is even greater for one who faces difficulty while fasting.

Make a Schedule

Making prayer priority, write down everything you want to accomplish that day. Chores, naptime, community service/charity and spiritual development are examples. At the end of each day, make a note of the next day's activities. Journal your progress to keep momentum and record your growth this Ramadan. There is a free download at ww.ProductiveMuslim.com called the Worksheet for Busy Moms from 2012.

Worship Smart, Not Hard

With a baby or toddler, you may not be able to sit for even 5 minutes without having to tend to them. Make Quran your background noise. The listener of Quran shares the reward with the reciter.

Every moment can turn into a moment of remembrance with words that are light on the tongue but heavy on the scales like SubhanAllah, Alhamdulillah, La illaha illAllah or Allahu Akbar.

It is that reported in the Hadith of 'Ali ibn Abi Taalib (Radi Allahu Anhu) who said that Fatimah (Radi Allahu Anha) came to the Prophet Muhammad (Sallallahu Alaihi Wasallam) and asked him for a servant. He said, "Shall I not tell you of something that is better for you than that? When you go to sleep, say 'Subhan'Allah' thirty-three times, 'Allhumdulillah' thirty-three times, and 'Allahu Akbar' thirty four times." (Sahih al-Bukhari 3113, Book 57, Hadith 22)

Dhikr to recite throughout the day:

Surah Ikhlaas

Reading this surah is equivalent to reading one third of the Quran.

"Narrated Abu Said Al-Khudri: A man heard another man reciting (Surah-Al-Ikhlas) 'Say He is Allah, (the) One.' (112. 1) repeatedly. The next morning he came to Allah's Messenger (pbuh) and informed him about it as if he thought that it was not enough to recite. On that Allah's Messenger (pbuh) said, "By Him in Whose Hand my life is, this Surah is equal to one-third of the Qur'an!" (Sahih al-Bukhari 5013, Book 66, Hadith 35)

Subhan'Allah wa biHamdihi *(Glory be to Allah and I Praise Him)*

Whoever says (the above) a hundred times during the day, his sins are wiped away, even if they are like the foam of the sea [Sahih al-Bukhari; 7:168, Muslim; 4:2071]

SubhanAllahi wa biHamdihi SubhanAllahil adheem *(Glory be to Allah, and Praise, Glory be to Allah, the Supreme)*

Prophet Muhammad (Sallallahu Alaihi Wasallam) said:

"Two words are light on the tongue, weigh heavily in the balance, they are loved by the Most Merciful One" [Sahih al-Bukhari; 7:67, Muslim; 4:2071]

Multiply Deeds

Multiply your deeds by giving some of your iftar meal to your neighbors or having family donate to a cause with you.
The Prophet Muhammad (saw) said:

"Whoever gives iftar to one who is fasting will have a reward like his, without that detracting from the reward of the fasting person in the slightest."

Cooking for your family is a source of blessing. With everthing you do, big or small, make intention to please Allah (swt). Transforming mundane activities to a form a worship is a way to stay engaged throughout the day. Rewards are multiplied by 70 this month.

Home Blessings

Unlike men who are obligated to attend prayers at the masjid, women are rewarded for praying at home. This privilege allows ease for mothers who care for young children. Dim the lights to help you focus, grab a mushaf, and pray with your children. Some nights, follow along with an online broadcast. You may find that this is a beautiful time to engage in worship as your baby drifts off to sleep.

If you know other families with young children, gather at a home once a week for a baby-friendly night of worship. When venturing out wear nursing-friendly clothing like an abaya with a zipper, button up jilbab or a loose tunic paired with a maxi skirt. Pack a nursing cover for easy, discreet nursing.

Small Deeds

Allah loves deeds that are regular, even if they are small. Do not push yourself to do more than you can handle. If one page of Quran a day is all you can do, that is okay. Give one dollar a day to charity. If you are too exhausted to stand for 20 rakats of tarawih, pray what you can. It is better to do some, than to abandon it. Find peace in knowing that your Lord loves you and will, inshAlah, forgive your sins.

The Prophet (Allah bless him & give him peace) is reported to have said:

> "Whoever stands in prayer in Ramadan, out of faith and seeking its reward, shall have all their past sins forgiven." [Bukhari, Muslim, Tirmidhi, and others]

Mommy's Helpers

Have friends and family help you a few times a week. They can watch the kids while you pray, study Quran or take a nap. If you know a sister who is menstruating or not fasting, she can helpout too!

Tarawih

Break up the prayer into five sets of 4 rakats. Take breaks in between to rest, eat, and tend to your children. If needed, recite short surahs to make each rakat brief. Tarawih can be finished in as little as 20 minutes.

Wear Your Baby

Sling babies cry less and nap more. They also have easier access to the breast. Latch and drape a nursing cover over them. A nursing necklace can be worn to entertain a busy child.

There are several types of carriers, but choose one that works best for you. A woven baby wrap or mei tai allows you to comfortably carry your child on your back, which will make prayer fun for the child. Ring slings are easily adjustable for nursing, plus the child can see moms face. Hip holders are great for a child who likes to look around. The website Nursengo.com sells a front/hip carrier that has a built in nursing cover.

A baby carrier is a necessity for busy parents. It creates less strain on the back and arms from holding a child multiple times a day. By distributing the child's weight and supporting good posture, baby-wearing prevents fatigue. Being hands-free allows the wearer to pray, read Quran, talk on the phone or multi-task while keeping their child content.

Nurse as Usual

Some mothers think they should make a feeding schedule or delay feedings so that the baby will eat less. This is not necessary and will lower milk supply. Also the child's weight and health could suffer from not getting enough nutrients. Breastfeed your child normally during Ramadan. Make sure they empty each breast so they get the higher calorie hindmilk. You may find that you have more milk at night because your body is digesting all the food and fluids from iftar. Also, prolactin levels are higher at night. To prevent your breasts from getting too full, you can wake your child to nurse or pump during these times.

Breast massage during nursing will help to increase milk production. Find a comfortable spot to nurse and pray each night. Use side lying and laidback positions so you can relax while nursing.

The most modest, practical nursing cover is the poncho/shawl style. These can be purchased online or handmade very easily with one yard of knit. Simply cut a small circle in the middle for your head.

Use a Two-Piece Prayer Garment

Buy a two-piece prayer garment that can be worn out the house for late night prayers. The long khimar (sleeves are a plus!) will make it easy to nurse in. Plus, they are loose and comfortable. Wear your baby over it in a sling. They will be calmer and quieter if they are close to you. You can pray while wearing them.

A French jilbab will work well, too. Some are designed with chest zippers, which makes nursing and babywearing even easier. I got mine from www.tasnimcollections.com years ago and still cherish it.

The best hijabs for nursing moms are maxi jersey, infinity and instant hijabs. No dangerous pins, fancy tricks or pulling.

Rest

A mid-day nap is essential. Exhaustion will hinder your productivity. Do not hesitate to break away from activities to allow your body and brain to refresh. Nursing is hard work that becomes a true jihad while fasting. If time allows take a power nap after iftar. You will feel much more energized later in the night if you take time to relax.

Nursing is meant to promote rest. Whenever a baby suckles the mother releases a hormone called cholecystokinin. This wonder causes her to relax and drift off to sleep. Breastmilk also calms the child. The reason many babies and toddlers nurse to sleep. Light activity will prevent the body from undue stress. As much as you may be driven join others, sit back and enjoy this phase. Taking a short walk with your family 1-2 hours after iftar is also relaxing.

Chapter 7

Get on Track: Start Eating Right

Breastmilk production can burn up to 500 calories a day. All nutrients needed for the child come from the mother's body. Therefore mindful eating is important. Drink plenty of water and fresh juice. Make fruits, vegetables, whole grains and nuts the majority of your intake. Cut out fast food and processed foods. Avoid unhealthy fats and sugars. Eat in moderation, stop eating before your stomach is full. Get in the habit of planning meals and grocery lists before shopping (especially while fasting). Start taking supplements, such as a prenatal vitamin, black seed, and probiotics daily.

Choose quality over quantity of foods. Metabolism becomes more efficient from fasting, meaning the body absorbs more nutrients. It will be helpful to use a juicer or high-powered blender like a Ninja. This will make it easier for you to take in extra fluids and nutrients. Drinks do not make you feel uncomfortably full like solid food. Especially if you have fasted all day, your stomach will tolerate this better. Green leafy vegetables and fruits go nicely in smoothies and juices. Save time by pre-packing ingredients in 30 bags before Ramadan starts. In the morning, take out one bag for your daily smoothie. Lastly, plan to eat a small midnight meal in addition to dinner and breakfast. Keep a food journal to log how much you drink and what foods you eat each day.

Suhoor

It's important that your body gets the calories and nutrients it needs to make milk. Set an alarm to avoid oversleeping as missing suhoor can have bad consequences, especially for the breastfeeding mom. Below are good foods to eat especially in the pre-dawn hours. Enjoy foods that restore your energy, increase milk production and keep your body hydrated.

Iftar

Eat iftar in two phases. Break the fast with dates and juice. Then have soup and salad. Soup is warm and gentle on the stomach. After prayers enjoy your main course. Split your plate into 1/4 protein, 1/4 carbs, and half vegetables.

Iftar provides 55% of the body's nutritional needs and restores blood sugar levels. Be careful not to overeat. Take it slow. Fresh fruit kebobs, black bean brownies, vegan ice cream (simply blend frozen bananas into a custard), or yogurt parfaits are great alternatives for a healthy dessert. Instead of coffee, enjoy a cup of herbal tea.

Dates

The best form of suhoor is dates as understood from the following hadith of the Prophet (saws), "How excellent are dates as the believer's suhoor." [(Sahih) Abu Dawood (2/303)]

Dates contains high levels of potassium, magnesium, B vitamins and fiber. This fruit will give your body a boost of energy.

Date Balls

Ingredients:

- 1 cup of raw, whole almonds

- 1 cup of fresh dates (or soak dried dates for 2 hrs prior to using)

- 1 tbsp natural peanut butter (or any nut butter)

- 3 tbsp coconut oil

- 3 tbsp cacao (or good quality cocoa)

- 2 tsp cinnamon

- 1 tbsp honey

Process the almonds until they are like crumbs. Add the rest of the ingredients and process until well combined. Using wet hands, roll the mixture into balls and place on a plate. Chill in the fridge for an hour to set.

Breakfast Bars

These can be enjoyed by the whole family.

- 3 cups old fashioned oatmeal

- 1/2 cup oat flour

- 1/4 cup flaxseed meal

- 1 cup sunflower seeds

- 1/4 cup brown sugar

- 1/2 cup honey

- 4 Tbsp. virgin organic coconut oil

- 1 Tbsp. vanilla flavor

- 1/4 tsp. sea salt

- 2 Cups Dried Cherries & Blueberries

- 3-4 Tbsp. Brewer's yeast (increases milk)

1. Preheat the oven to 400 degrees Fahrenheit.

2. Prepare a 15-inch x 10-inch baking dish by lining it with parchment paper. Spray it with nonstick cooking spray.

3. In a large bowl mix the oats, oat flour, flaxseed meal and sunflower seeds.

4. Pour the mixture onto a baking dish (not the one you just prepared). Bake for 10-15 minutes or until golden brown. Stir to make sure it cooks evenly.

5. Remove mixture from the oven and carefully pour back into the bowl. Stir in dried fruit and brewer's yeast. Set aside.

6. In a saucepan, mix brown sugar, honey, coconut oil and vanilla. Over medium heat, stirring constantly, bring to a simmer. Remove from heat.

7. Pour sugar/honey mixture over oat mixture in the large bowl, be careful, the mixture is very hot. Mix very well, making sure to coat all ingredients evenly.

8. Pour the granola mixture into your prepared baking dish, on top of the parchment paper. Spread out the mixture with a spatula.

9. Now fold over the sides of the parchment paper or add a sheet on top, and press down firmly all over the granola.

10. Let the granola cool for 2 hours.

11. Remove the top parchment paper and carefully place granola onto a large cutting board, peeling away the rest of the paper.

12. Cut granola into bars with a large knife by firmly pressing down.

Barley Porridge- Talbinah

This yogurt-like dish was enjoyed by the Prophet (pbuh) and his companions. Aishah often had it prepared for sick or grieving people. The Messenger (sallallaahu alayhi wasallam) also said: "The talbina gives rest to the heart of the patient and makes it active and relieves some of his sorrow and grief." Saheeh al-Bukhaaree (5325). Barley is known to be good for heart disease, depression and diabetics. It is high in beta glucan and tryptophan which both increase prolactin levels in the blood. It also contains B vitamins, iron, magnesium, zinc, phosphorus, copper, and is one of the richest sources of chromium, which is important in maintaining blood glucose levels.

Ingredients:

- 100% whole grain barley flour

- Milk/Coconut milk

- Water

- Honey

1. Pour 2 tablespoons of barley flour into 2 cups of water or milk (you can do half water half milk).

2. Stir on low heat for about 10-15 minutes or until a porridge-like consistency is reached. Add water if needed to thin.

3. Sweeten with honey.

Fresh Fruit

Prepare a fruit salad and refrigerate the night before to save time. Dried fruits are also a healthy alternative. For example figs, mango, coconut, apricots or prunes. The best fruits for nursing moms include green papaya (unripe), apricots, bananas, strawberries, cantaloupe, avocado, sapodilla, grapefruit, and blueberries.

Green Smoothie

Green foods increase the fat content of breastmilk and will give you an energy boost. Collards, spinach, kale, wheat grass, or any other green leafy vegetables can be juiced or chopped into smoothies. Spirulina, kelp, barley grass, alfalfa leaf and herbs are also great green foods to add to your morning drink. Save your greens from going bad by blending a bunch of greens with a bit of water. Pour into ice cube tray and freeze. When frozen, pop green cubes into a freezer bag. Add a few cubes to your morning smoothie with a mix of fruit and a liquid base.

I love to add chia seeds which are high in omega-3 fatty acids to my smoothies. A few spoonfuls of flax powder provides fiber that helps prevent constipation. The following recipe contains moringa, the most nutrient dense plant in the world. It treats many diseases and is a well known milk booster. The leaves contain:

- 7 times the Vitamin C content of oranges

- 4 times the calcium content of milk

- 4 times the vitamin content of carrots

- 3 times the potassium content of bananas

- 2 times the protein found in yogurt

Moringa Smoothie

- 2-4 leaves of kale or chard

- 1 banana

- 1 Tbsp. almond butter

- 1 date

- ½ - ¾ cups coconut water

- 1 Tbsp. cacao powder

- 1 tsp. moringa leaf

- 1 cup ice

Place all smoothie ingredients in a high speed blender and blend until smooth.

Eggs

Eggs are a great source of protein and omega 3 fatty acids. Eggs can also be baked into a quiche or frittata. If boiled eggs are too bland for you, boil them the night before and make an egg salad. Egg curry is a good dish also. They are also more flavorful if you sprinkle dukkah an Egyptian spice, and a drizzle of olive oil on top.

Oats

Oats are the most commonly used food to increase milk supply in the U.S. It is one of the most nutritious foods and contains proteins, vitamins, minerals, and trace elements. Save time by mixing raw oats and water or milk the night before and placing the bowl in the refrigerator. In the morning it will be thickened and can be eaten cold or warm. You can also easily prepare old-fashioned cut oatmeal in a slow cooker the night before suhoor. Stir in dried fruits, nuts, spices, milk and butter for a boost of nutrients. Oats can also be prepared in advance as granola or breakfast bars. Broken wheat is another option that can be made into porridge. Muesli, a mix of oats, nuts and dried fruit is available in many middle eastern stores.

Oatcakes Recipe

Prepare two dozen and store for the week's early morning meals. This recipe makes 12 oatcakes.

- 3 cups rolled oats

- 2 cups whole wheat pastry flour

- 1/4 tsp baking powder

- 2 tsp salt cup

- 1/2 flax seeds

- 3/4 cup chopped walnuts, lightly toasted

- 1/3 cup coconut oil

- 3/4 cup maple syrup

- 1/2 cup sugar

- 2 large eggs, lightly beaten

Preheat oven to 325° F. Grease a 12 cup muffin pan. Mix oats, flour, baking powder, salt flax seeds and walnuts in a large bowl. Put a medium saucepan on low heat. Add coconut oil, butter, maple syrup, and sugar. Slowly melt until sugar just dissolves and butter melts. Avoid getting it too hot. Pour the mixture into the large bowl with the oat mixture. Stir together until wet dough forms. Spoon dough into muffin cups until nearly full. Bake 25-30 minutes, or until edges are golden. Remove pan from oven and let cool for 5 minutes. Run a knife along edge of the cakes and tip them out to finish cooling.

Overnight Oats

Make this recipe ahead of time for a convenient breakfast or late night snack. Mason jars work well for this recipe.

- 1/2 cup old fashion rolled oats

- 1/2 cup milk

- 1 tablespoon plain yogurt

- 1/2 teaspoon honey

- 1 tablespoon raisins

- 1/8 teaspoon vanilla

- 2 to 3 pinches cinnamon

Mix together all ingredients, cover, and refrigerate for a minimum of 5 hours before eating. Alternatively mix in an insulated thermos container (left unrefrigerated) and wait no more than 7 hours before eating. Enjoy chilled or microwave for 30 -60 seconds.

Mama's Oatmeal

This warm bowl of goodness, is full of ingredients that support lactation.

- 1 cup old fashioned rolled oats (not instant)

- 2 cups water

- 1/3 cup unsweetened coconut flakes

- 1 scoop chia seeds

- 3 tbsp. ground flax seeds

- 1-2 tsp blackstrap molasses - a source of iron

- 1 tbsp. almond butter

- 1 ripe banana, sliced

- 1 tsp maple syrup

- pinch of sea salt

Bring the oatmeal and water to a boil for a minute. Reduce the heat and let simmer. As it thickens, add the coconut, flax, chia, almond butter, banana and salt. Stir well.

Once fully thickened to your liking, stir in the blackstrap molasses and maple syrup.

Serve with milk of your choice.

Hummus

Chickpeas are known to increase milk supply. Also, the sesame seed butter or tahini is a strong source of calcium. I highly recommend making your own hummus because it is less expensive and tastes better. For an extra boost of nutrients to your milk supply, add raw or roasted garlic. Make a wrap by spreading it on thin flatbread or tortillas. Add chopped vegetables, roll tightly and refrigerate until ready to eat.

Baked Yams

Baked yams can be prepared the previous night and eaten cold or warmed in the morning. Sprinkle with a little brown sugar and butter for extra flavor.

Meat

A small serving of meat in the morning can make you feel more energized. Meat takes 16 hours to digest and provides sustained energy. It contains heme iron that is 15% more digestive than plant iron. It helps plant iron to absorb better so eat it in combination with vegetables. For example an omelet muffin (simply mix 8 eggs with 8 ounces of cooked meat and few chopped vegetables. Season with a little salt & pepper and add 2 tablespoons of water/milk. Pour into greased muffin tins or parchment paper cups. Bake at 350° degrees F for 18 minutes or until set. Fresh halal meat is best like lamb or shredded chicken. Avoid processed products like hotdogs, frozen chicken patties and canned corn beef.

Lentil Soup

Make a pot of soup to last a few days. Add fennel to increase your milk supply. Mung beans and fava beans (foul) are great alternatives.

Nuts

Nuts are great for suhoor because they require no preparation. Almonds, macadamia nuts, and cashews are also known to support milk supply. Make a mix and keep it on the dining room table.

Chia Seed Pudding

In some traditional cultures, chia seeds were used as an energy food. It contains as much calcium as a glass of milk, more Omega-3s than a serving of walnuts and as many antioxidants as blueberries. The small seed absorbs lots of liquid which helps to prevent dehydration. Enjoy this rich, creamy pudding.

- 6 large Mejdool dates, pitted (soak in water if hard)
- 1 cup of cold milk
- 2 Tablespoons to 4 Tablespoons of cocoa powder
- 1 teaspoon of vanilla
- 3 tablespoons of chia seeds

Place everything in the blender on high speed until the pudding is smooth and perfectly thickened.

Bone Broth

Traditional bone broth is inexpensive to make and very nourishing for breastfeeding moms. It is simmered for a long time, so prepare it in advance or keep a pot boiling during the week. Just add water as needed. Bone broth is high in minerals, especially calcium, phosphorus and magnesium. These are important for the baby to grow healthy, strong bones. If these nutrients are not in your diet, your body will take them from your own bones and give them to baby. For this reason bone broth helps to prevent bone density loss by replenishing your stores.

The body absorbs the minerals in bone broth easier than in supplements. Bone broth also naturally contains gelatin. The collagen in this is good for skin, hair and nail growth. It supports joints and connective tissue. It contains two key nutrients glucosamine and chondroitin for joint care. Also, it's a good source of amino acids, the building blocks of protein. These help to boost the immune system, promote sleep and calm the mind, improve digestion and fight inflammation.

Bone broth also calms the stomach and soothes nausea. Use two or more pounds of leftover bones from meals or goto a halal butchery and ask for bones. They are usually very cheap and sometimes free. You can use raw bones with or without the meat and skin. You can also use extra scrap vegetables from a previous meal. You will need a slow cooker or a large pot and a fine strainer.

Directions:

1. Roast the bones on 350°F for 30 minutes to improve final taste. Place bones in pot and cover with cool water and 1/4 cup of apple cider vinegar or lemon juice. Let sit for 30 minutes. This helps to leach the minerals.

2. Coarsely chop vegetables such as carrot, onion, or celery and add them to the pot.

3. Add spices, salt, pepper or herbs as you like.

4. Bring broth to a boil and then turn it low to simmer. There should be a gentle, slow bubbling. Watch for a thin film that floats to the top in the first two hours. Remove it with a large spoon.

5. Check the pot periodically and add water if it is low.

6. Add fresh vegetables or herbs in the last hour if you want to make it like a soup. It is recommended to simmer lamb, beef or bison for 8-72 hours. Poultry for 8-24 hours. Fish heads and bones for 6-24 hours.

7. When the broth is ready, turn off the heat and let it cool. Strain it. The bones and bits can be thrown out.

The broth can be kept in the fridge for 5 days or froze for later. It can be used to sauté vegetables, make soups, gravies and sauces. Or, you can add a dash of salt and sip it like tea. Drink at least a cup a day.

Whole Wheat Pancakes

Again, these can be prepared the night before and served cold or warm. Add flaxseed to your batter for extra nutrients, especially omega-3 fatty acids.

- 4 cups milk

- 3 1/2 tbsp apple cider vinegar

- 1 tsp baking soda

- 3 large eggs

- 1 tsp salt

- 2 3/4 cups whole wheat flour

- 2 3/4 cups whole rolled oats

- 1 cup flax seed

- 1/2 cup nutritional yeast

- 1/4 cup honey

- 2 tsp cinnamon

- 1 tsp vanilla

Directions

1. Preheat griddle to 325° F.

2. Measure milk into large bowl; add vinegar and allow to stand for 10 minutes.

3. Lightly hand-beat eggs with honey and vanilla; add to milk mixture and mix.

4. Combine dry ingredients in another bowl.

5. Add milk and egg mixture to dry ingredients. Mix well.

6. On hot griddle, pour 1/3 cup of batter for each pancake.

7. Cook on one side until edges are dry and center is bubbly.

8. Flip and cook until underside is medium brown color.

9. Serve topped with pastured butter, nut butters, fresh or pureed fruits, pure maple syrup, raw honey, or other toppings.

Storage:

Store extra cakes in the refrigerator for breakfasts throughout the week or store in the freezer for up to three months.

Muffins

Nearly anything can be made into a muffin. Incorporate vegetables, fruits, grains or nuts into a basic recipe. Oatmeal-raisin and morning glory muffins are two of my favorites. They store easily and are always ready to eat. The following recipe will boost milk supply and is full of nutrients.

Pumpkin Chocolate Muffins

- 2 eggs

- ½ cup honey

- 1 cup pureed pumpkin

- ½ cup melted coconut or grapeseed oil

- ½ cup unsweetened applesauce

- 1 teaspoon vanilla

- 1 cup whole wheat flour

- ⅔ cup almond flour

- 1 teaspoon baking soda

- ½ teaspoon salt

- ½ teaspoon baking powder

- ½ cup chopped walnuts

- ⅓ cup chocolate chips plus extra to top muffins (or dried fruit like raisins or cranberries)

- 2 tablespoons chia seeds

- 3 tablespoons flaxseed meal

- 2 tablespoons brewer's yeast

Preheat oven to 350 degrees F. Whisk together the wet ingredients. In another bowl, combine the dry ingredients (whole wheat flour through brewer's yeast). Add the dry ingredients to the wet and mix well. Line muffin tins with paper. Fill each to the top with batter and top with chocolate chips (optional). Bake 25 to 30 minutes for regular muffins, 22 minutes for mini muffins, and 55 minutes for a loaf. They are ready with toothpick inserted in the middle comes out clean. Cool for a few minutes in the pan on a rack.

Water

While it is not "food" per se, water it is extremely important. Without proper hydration, any attempt at fasting will be difficult and dangerous. Balance your water-food intake at suhoor. You don't want to drink so much water that you end up urinating excessively til you simply flush your system instead of hydrating it. Nor do you want to fill yourself up before getting the required nutrients from your meal. Instead, be conscious of your fluid intake starting at Maghrib and moderately drink throughout the night. Mothers need about 2-3 liters a day. Your body will retain fluids better if you sip your water as opposed to gulping it down. Keep a water bottle just for youself always filled and keep it in your bag when you go out. You can make flavored waters with herbs, black seeds, and fruits e.g. lemons, mint, or cucumbers. Chill at least a a gallon of water in the fridge with your favorite add-ins.

Smart tip: Buy a large beverage dispenser with a built-in fruit infuser. There will always be plenty to share and keep you satisfied.

Recommendations:

1. Drink Zam Zam water whenever you can. It is very nutritious and pure. Due to it's alkaline nature, it reduces acid in the stomach which prevents heartburn.

2. Adding a little apple cider vinegar to your water has many benefits.

3. Coconut water is an excellent source of electrolytes and is a great rehydrating beverage. It is very similar in composition to blood plasma. Young coconuts can have up to a pint of water. Crack these open and drain them in the evening.

4. Aloe vera juice is also very hydrating.

5. Fennel/barley water is a tried-and-true remedy for boost milk production. Soak a half cup pearled barley in three cups cold

water overnight, or boil the barley and water for 25 minutes. Strain out barley. Store barley water in refrigerator or cool place until needed. Then heat a cup or two to boiling and add fennel seeds—one teaspoon per cup of barley water. Steep for no longer than 30 minutes. This drink also helps with digestion. If you do not have time to do this, add Ovaltine to a glass of milk each night. It contains barley.

Rosehip Electrolyte Drink

by Ameera Rahim

- dried rosehips

- 1 cup orange juice

- ¼ cup lemon juice

- 1/8 teaspoon Himalayan salt

- 2 cup coconut water

- 1 tablespoon honey or more

1. Pour one cup of boiling water over 1 tbs of dried rosehips, cover and let steep for 30-60 mins.

2. Strain out the rosehips herbs (discard them) and then combine the rosehips tea with the rest of the ingredients to have your homemade herbal electrolyte drink.

Great for hot summer days and when you're not feeling well. Each ingredient serves a beneficial immune boosting purpose and replenishes your body's energy.

Super Juice

Juice one beet, two carrots, a quarter of a lemon and half a fennel bulb. This combo is good for the liver and immune system. Plus, it increases milk.

Oils & Butters

Use these to prepare or drizzle on your meals. They contain good fats. Coconut, olive, grape seed, flaxseed and sesame are all healthy oils. Use butter or ghee in moderation. These help to boost your energy.

Nut Milk

Make your own almond milk. It's easy and costs less than buying it from the store. All you need is a blender and strainer. Soak one cup of almonds for up to 12 hours. Blend with 4 cups of water then strain. Put back in blender with a date for sweetness and vanilla. Blend and drink.

Tumeric Paste

Tumeric is has many health benefits including anti-inflammatory, antioxidant, aids digestion and boosts the immune system.

- ½ tsp black pepper

- 1 tsp ginger powder

- ½ tsp cinnamon

- ½ tsp cardamom

- ¼ tsp salt

- ½ cup turmeric powder

- 1½ cups water, plus ½ cup more

- ½ cup coconut oil and/or ghee

- ¼ cup raw honey

1. Combine pepper, ginger, cinnamon, cardamom, and salt in a small bowl. Set aside.

2. Combine turmeric and 1 and ½ cups of water in a small pot, stirring constantly with a wooden spoon. Bring mixture to a very gentle simmer and add another ½ cup of water.

3. Continue to stir with wooden spoon. Add mixed spices and continue to cook and stir on low for 3 minutes, until you have a thick and smooth paste.

4. Turn off heat and add oil or ghee. Continue to stir until completely smooth.

5. Cool and transfer to clean glass jar. Mixture will thicken as it cools. Place lid on jar after mixture has completely cooled.

6. Give a little shake to prevent separation and store in fridge for 2 weeks.

7. Add one teaspoon to a cup of warm milk for golden milk.

Nursing Tea

Have a cup of herbal tea that supports breastmilk production. If you prefer to make your own try this recipe for cold tea:

- 1 gallon of water

- 1 tablespoon of Fennel Seeds

- 1/2 tablespoon of Dill Seeds

- 1 tablespoon of Fenugreek Seeds

1. Boil the water

2. Mix together the Fennel, Dill and Fenugreek seeds

3. Add the seeds to the boiling water and boil on medium for 30 minutes until the tea is nice and brown. Sweeten with honey if you like.

4. Let the tea cool

5. Fill recycled water bottles with tea and store in refrigerator. Drink a bottle daily.

Breastfeeding Bread

Ingredients

- Soft butter, for greasing your loaf pan

For the bread dough:

- 1 teaspoon aniseed

- 1 teaspoon caraway seeds

- 1 teaspoon fennel seeds

- 1 teaspoon fenugreek

- 4 1/8 cups or 500g strong wholemeal spelt flour

- 7g fast-acting dried yeast

- 2 teaspoons sea salt flakes

- 1/4 cup or 50g pine nuts of which: 1 tablespoon set aside

- 1/4 cup or 50g pumpkin seeds of which: 1 tablespoon set aside

- 1/4 cup or 50g sunflower seeds of which: 1 tablespoon set aside

- 3 tablespoons or 45ml extra virgin olive oil

- 1 1/2 cups or 350ml warm water

For the egg wash:

- 1 egg

- Splash of water

Method

1. Grease your bread pan generously with softened butter and set aside, along with your one tablespoon of each pine nuts, pumpkin seeds and sunflower seeds for decorating.

2. Grind your spices with a mortar and pestle or a spice grinder.

3. Mix all of your dry ingredients in the bowl of your stand mixer or in a bowl large enough to knead the dough in.

4. Add in the oil and mix well.

5. Add in the warm water and mix again.

6. Knead with your bread hook or by hand in your bowl for just a few minutes, until smooth.

7. Dough will be sticky but add flour as needed.

8. Scrape the dough out of the bowl and use damp hands to shape it into a loaf . Put in loaf pan.

9. Whisk the egg with a splash of water to create an egg wash.

10. Cut some slashes into the top of the dough and then brush it with your egg wash.

11. Sprinkle on the reserved seeds and nuts, tapping them down gently so they stick.

12. Place in a large plastic bag in warm place and leave to rise until doubled.

13. When your dough is nearly ready, preheat your oven to 450°F.

14. Bake the bread for the first 20 minutes, then turn the oven down to 400°F for an additional 15-20 minutes. Cover with foil if your toppings look like they might begin to scorch.

15. Turn out to cool on a wire rack.

Lactogenic Foods

- Vegetables- Fennel root, beetroot, carrots, yam, sweet potato, dark leafy greens like kale, spinach, romaine lettuce and mustard greens

- Fruit- Dates, Figs, Apricots, Green papaya, Goji Berries

- Good Fats- Butter, Olive Oil, Coconut Oil Flaxseed Oil, Sesame Oil (Be sure to get plenty of fats) – supplement with fish oil and evening primrose oil.

- Grains- Barley, Oats/Oatmeal, Quinoa, Rice, Millet, Buckwheat

- Nuts and Seeds- Almonds, Sesame Seed, Sunflower Seed, Chia Seed, Hemp Seed, Flaxseed, Coconut Legumes Chickpeas, Lentils, Peas, Green beans, Adzuki, Kidney, Black or White Beans

- Animal Products Choose Organic, antibiotic- free, full fat meat and dairy, wild caught small fish

- Herbs/Spices: Marjoram, Basil, Pepper, Fennel, Anise, Dill, Caraway, Cumin, Dandelion

- Condiments: Garlic, Ginger, Onion

- Avoid Large Amounts: Parsley, Sage, Rosemary, Thyme, Peppermint

Chapter 8

Is My Baby Getting Enough?

It's normal to be concerned about your milk supply. Your child's well being is priority. Many women mistake softer breasts, a fussy baby or more frequent nursing as a sign that their milk is gone. But your milk supply is okay if your baby is urinating and stooling normally. Obviously their growth pattern should also be consistent. A growth spurt, teething or other changes in routine such as going to the mosque at night will change your child's nursing patterns. It is normal for them to nurse more often, longer or even shorter. If you have concerns go to a breastfeeding expert or clinic to get help.

If you or your child are showing signs of poor milk supply, stop fasting and rest. Remember Allah (swt) has allowed you to make up these fasts. This condition is temporary. Your child is growing and will be weaned in two years.

Allah burdens not a person beyond his scope. (Surah Al Baqarah, Verse 286)

Enjoy this special bond, there is no better substitute! Nurse your baby on demand, do skin to skin conact and drink lots of fluids to increase your milk.

The Signs

1. Your baby's weight: The best measure of whether your baby is getting enough milk is his or her weight gain. If you are concerned about your milk supply, have your baby weighed and re-weighed using the same baby scale. Have a lactation consultant evaluate them, keeping in mind that there may be slight variations due to mothers temporary diet changes.   A home scale can used every 10 days at the least, if you are super concerned. It is not necessary to weigh them everyday.

2. Diaper output: You can get a sense of how much your baby is taking in by what comes out. Your child should have at least five very wet diapers per day. Pale, odorless urine is normal. Their stools may vary. For example, some babies stool three times a week. Other may go four times a day, it is all normal. Stools should be larger if days have passed. Diapers will show soft, greenish-yellow, seedy poop. It is also normal to see variations of orange, brown, and yellow which reflect the gut juices and bile that digest milk. It can be creamy or like a paste. Any formula, supplements or food will change the color and consistency. Usually thicker, smelly and multicolored with bits of undigested food. But if your child starts pooping less, becomes fussy, straining or pushing pebble like turds, they are constipated. This is most often caused by starting solids, especially cereal, and formula. Try giving them one ounce of water, prune, pear or apple juice a few times a day. Plums, apricots, peaches, broccoli, brown rice and avocado are gentler foods to digest.

3. Audible swallowing: A period of swallowing during a feeding shows that your baby is getting milk. To check for swallowing, listen for a 'cah' sound, squeak or gulp, and look for a longer and slower movement of the jaw, often with a brief pause at the widest point. The breasts usually become fuller after breaking the fast. If your child drinks less during the day when you are fasting, you should have more active feeds later.

4. Appearance & Behavior: Your child should be alert and active. They should have supple skin that has a healthy, normal color.

To ensure they get the most milk offer both breasts each feed, burping in between each. Keep them on the breast for 10-20 minutes. Older babies tend to eat much quicker. Nurse 8 times in 24 hours or whatever is normal for your child. Allow the child to fall asleep or come of the breast naturally.

Soft Breasts

As your body adjust to taking in less fluid and food during daytime hours your milk production will slow down. You can still make enough to sustain your child by nursing throughout the day and night. Expect fuller breasts 1-2 hours after breaking your fast. A letdown may even occur while you are breaking your fast, as your bood sugar spikes. Your body will re-adjust your milk supply, increasing after the initial dip to meet your child's needs.

Fussy Evenings

It is common for babies to be fussy in the evening. Frustration can rise when mom is in the last hours of fasting. Depending on your child's temperament, they can be just as frustrated with all the changes in Ramadan. Get help in the evenings, or use a sling to calm them. Make sure dinner is started early in a slow cooker, so you can relax in the last few hours. This is often the toughest part of the day. Massage can be used to calm them. Distraction is a great way to redirect a toddler. Have an early bath time. Provide them with a cup or popsicle of breastmilk. Make sure they nap one or twice earlier in the day to prevent a meltdown at maghrib. Have quiet after nap by reading a book or doing puzzles (no electronics).

Supplementing

If needed supplement with expressed breastmilk. Use a Medela Softfeeder or small cup. A baby can drink from a cup as long as you support them and pace the feeding. Bottles should be avoided to prevent nipple confusion and breast refusal. It's important to keep your child latching! Do lots of skin to skin contact, and take a break from fasting so that your body will produce more milk. Always offer the breast before supplementing.

If you have no more extra, stored breastmilk, ask fellow sisters if they would like to be your child's milk mother by donating milk or co-nursing. Human milk from another woman is much healthier and safer than formula, contrary to popular belief. Plus, wet-nursing is a sunnah.

If this isn't possible checkout an informed milk sharing network like Human Milk for Human Babies.

Alternatively you could buy a halal certified baby formula. Look for an "M", halal or kosher symbol. Call the company if unsure of ingredients. Always prepare formula according to the package directions.

If non-human milk is used, changes in the baby's gut flora occur and will cause changes in the frequency, odor and consistency of baby's stool. They will also settle differently after feeds. For example, they may be more fussy or gassy. In order to reduce the likelihood of an adverse reaction, the baby who has a family history of allergies should not be exposed to non-human milk if possible.

Homemade infant formula recipe

Some mothers choose to make their own formula to avoid GMOs, chemicals and additives. Children with allergies and stomach issues often do well with homemade formula. This is not meant to completely replace mother's milk.

- 4 cups homemade coconut milk or use rice, hemp, almond or organic cow's milk

- 2-4 tbsp Brown rice protien (start with 1, then increase if no constipation)

- 1 tbsp Blackstrap molasses

- 1 tbsp Pediatrivite, liquid infant multivitamin

- 1/4 tsp Infant probiotic powder

- 1/2 tsp Cod liver oil

- 2 tbsp Flax seed, coconut or hemp oil

- 1 drop of infant, 400 IU Vitamin D

Mix all ingredients in a Magic-bullet or other good blender. Store in refrigerator for 48 hours in a glass container, then discard unused milk.

Baby Tracker

Day	# of Wet Diapers 5+	Stool? yes/no	# of Breastfeeds 8+	Supplement? How much?
1				
2				
3				
4				
5				
6				
7				
8				
9				
10				
11				
12				
13				
14				
15				
16				
17				
18				
19				
20				
21				
22				
23				
24				
25				
26				
27				
28				
29				
30				

Am I Too Dehydrated?

Any combination of these symptoms is your body telling you that it is not getting enough fluids. Be on the lookout for these and seek medical attention when necessary. Usually a day or two of rest resolves everything. Re-assess your situation and decide what's best for you- continuing to fast may not be the best choice.

- Constipation

- Vomiting

- Very little/dark urine

- Dizziness

- Dry mouth

- Fatigue

- Headaches

For more info on fasting while nursing:
visit www.ramadanfastingandpregnancy.wordpress.com

Studies on Fasting and Breastfeeding

- Mazidi M, Rezaie P, Nematy M. The Effects of Ramadan Fasting on Growth Parameters: A Narrative Review. Journal of Fasting and Health. 2014;2(1):41-45.

- Haratipour H, Sohrabi MB, Ghasemi E, Karimi A, Zolfaghari P, Yahyaei E. Impact of maternal fasting during Ramadan on growth parameters of exclusively breastfed infants in Shahroud, 2012. Journal of Fasting and Health. 2013;1(2):66-69.

- Bajaj S, Khan A, Fathima FN, et al. South Asian consensus statement on women's health and Ramadan. Indian J Endocrinol Metab. 2012;16(4):508-11.

- Kridli SA. Health beliefs and practices of Muslim women during Ramadan. MCN Am J Matern Child Nurs. 2011 Jul-Aug;36(4):216-21; quiz 222-3.

- Zimmerman DR, Goldstein L, Lahat E, Braunstein R, Stahi D, Bar-Haim A, Berkovitch M. Effect of a 24+ hour fast on breast milk composition. J Hum Lact. 2009 May;25(2):194-8.

- Khodel A, Kheiri S, Nasiri J, Taheri E, Najafi M, Salehifard A, Jafari A. Comparison of Growth Parameters of Infants of Ramadan Fasted and Non-Fasted Mothers. Iranian Journal of Endocrinology and Metabolism. 2008;10(2):155-161.

- Khoshdel A, Najafi M, Kheiri S, Taheri E, Nasiri J, Yousofi H, Jafari A. Impact of Maternal Ramadan Fasting on Growth Parameters in Exclusively Breast-fed Infants. Iranian Journal of Pediatrics 2007. 17(4):345-352.

- Rashid H. Ramadan Fasting And Breast Milk. Breastfeeding Medicine. 2007 Mar;2(1):59-60. doi:10.1089/bfm.2006.0021.

- Rakicioğlu N, Samur G, Topçu A, Topçu AA. The effect of Ramadan on maternal nutrition and composition of breast milk. Pediatr Int. 2006 Jun;48(3):278-83.

- Tigas S, Sunehag A, Haymond MW. Metabolic adaptation to feeding and fasting during lactation in humans. J Clin Endocrinol Metab. 2002 Jan;87(1):302-7.

- Beneremail A, Galadari S, Gillett M, Osman N, Al-Taneiji H, Al-Kuwaiti MHH, Al-Sabosy MMA. Fasting during the holy month of Ramadan does not change the composition of breast milk. Nutrition Research. 2001Jun;21(6):859-864.

- Ertem IO, Kaynak G, Kaynak C, Ulukol B, Gulnar SB. Attitudes and practices of breastfeeding mothers regarding fasting in Ramadan. Child Care Health Dev. 2001 Nov;27(6):545-54.

- Neville MC, Sawicki VS, Hay WW Jr. Effects of fasting, elevated plasma glucose and plasma insulin concentrations on milk secretion in women. J Endocrinol. 1993 Oct;139(1):165-73.

- Hamosh M, Dewey KG, Garza C, et al: Nutrition During Lactation. Institute of Medicine, Washington, DC, National Academy Press, 1991, p. 92. This book is available free from the HRSA Information Center.

- Neville M, Oliva-Rasbach J. Is maternal milk production limiting for infant growth during the first year of life in breast-fed infants? p. 123-133 in Goldman AS, Atkinson SA, Hanson LA, eds. Human Lactation 3: The Effects of Human Milk on the the Recipient Infant. Plenum Press 1987, New York.

- Prentice AM, Lamb WH, Prentice A, Coward WA. The effect of water abstention on milk synthesis in lactating women. Clin Sci (Lond). 1984 Mar;66(3):291-8.

- Prentice AM, Prentice A, Lamb WH, Lunn PG, Austin S. Metabolic consequences of fasting during Ramadan in pregnant and lactating women. Hum Nutr Clin Nutr. 1983 Jul;37(4):283-94.

Chapter 9

Pumping

Are you exclusively pumping, a student or a working mom? Here are a few tips to help you while pumping outside of the home:

- Be consistent! This will help to maintain your milk supply.

- Make a routine for pumping at work or home. Set the time, place, chair, etc. Prepare your equipment the same way each day.

- Let your boss know that it is Ramadan! Provide them with a resource such as The Working Muslim in Ramadan Guide for Employers published by Working Muslim.

- Pump at night or in the early morning. Pumping between iftar and suhoor will ensure you get good output.

- If you pump during the day and notice a dip in your supply, set aside time to pump after you have regained your energy from eating and drinking.

- Upgrade to a hospital grade pump. Mothers usually express more milk and maintain their supply more efficiently with these powerful pumps.

- Nurse on demand when you are with your child.

- Avoid skipping nursing or pumping sessions, even if your supply looks like it's lowering.

- Get plenty of rest.

- Take a supplement to increase your milk supply such as fenugreek.

- Jiggle, shake and roll your breast for one minute before pumping.

- Homeopathic Rescue Remedy can be used to relax you and stimulate letdown

- Do not look at the bottles while pumping. Relax and listen or watch something.

- Use a double pump instead of a single. Double pumping yields more milk.

- Massage or do compression on your breasts while pumping. This will make more milk come out.

- Re-hydrate overnight. Make sure you are drinking enough fluids when you are not fasting.

- Avoid overeating. Keep yourself cool and pace yourself.

- Eat a well-balanced diet with many fruits and vegetables. Try juicing or making smoothies to get adequate nutrients.

- Keep a few things that remind you of your child in your bag such as photos, a shirt, toy or recording of them. This will help you relax and encourage let-down while you are pumping.

- Prepare and pack your supplies (storage bags, breast pads, clean bottles, cool packs etc.) at night or before suhoor.

- Use a pumping bustier so you can relax while pumping. This bra will hold the flanges connected to the bottles, making pumping hands-free.

Chapter 10

25 Ways to Prevent Burnout

Breastfeeding research tells us that short term fasting will not decrease milk supply, but that severe dehydration can reduce milk supply. A nursing woman may be at risk of severe dehydration if she is not drinking enough fluids during the night period. This risk will be heightened if she is exhausted with the demands of work, homemaking, caregiving and other daytime activities. Succumbed to too much physical and emotional stress, a breastfeeding mother can easily become burned-out while fasting. ProducingbBreastmilk takes 25% of the body's energy. Consequently, many Muslimahs blame fasting during Ramadan as the reason they stopped breastfeeding. It saddens me that such an exciting time of the year, hinders women from providing the best nourishment for their children. As mentioned in the Surah Al-Baqarah verse 233, breastfeeding should not be a hardship.

As a community, we should take more efforts to support women who are fasting, especially during Ramadan. Essential to maintaining well-being, proper rest, a healthy diet, strong support network and remembrance of Allah will ensure mothers enjoy the barakah of breastfeeding and fasting. Please share the following tips to help mothers protect their health and milk supply this Ramadan:

1. Avoid caffeinated and/or carbonated drinks such as soda, coffee and tea which can cause dehydration. Caffeine is a diuretic which means it increases urination.

2. Eat fresh fruits and vegetable as much as you can.

3. Recite Quran daily to help you relax.

4. Do not fill-up on food at suhoor. Set a schedule (if it helps) and eat in moderation overnight.

5. Complete housework at night or before suhoor.

6. Avoid spicy foods.

7. Make dhikr throughout the day to keep you busy and focused.

8. Protect yourself from overheating by wearing hats, shades and light clothing when outside the house.

9. Build a support network with sisters who are also mothers.

10. Take a break from cooking by inviting others over for pot-luck style iftar and/or attending community iftars

11. Limit your intake of dairy products like milk, cheese and yogurt because they contribute to mucous production (thickening of body fluids).

12. If you work outside the home, sit down and rest in between high activity flows.

13. Though it may be a challenge, find time to be alone. Journal, meditate or reflect. Stress can lower milk supply, so find a way to relax.

14. Discuss your intention to fast with your husband, family and friends before fasting, to avoid negative feedback.

15. Ask family and friends for help with housework, children, cooking, etc.

16. Plan activities for children to keep them busy during the day. For example, Islamic DVDs, games or crafts.

17. Make a list for grocery shopping and plan your meals weekly.

18. Break your fast with a cup of juice or water and 3-4 dates to bring your blood sugar levels to normal.

19. Make dua to Allah (swt), calling him by his glorious name Ar-Razzaq (The Provider), to provide you with the strength to continue fasting. Remember to give salawat to the Prophet Muhammad (saws) in your dua.

20. Recite Ayat-ul-Kursi. There are many benefits to reading this verse.

21. Recite Surah Al-Ikhlas and Al-Mu'awwidhatain. In a Hadith, Abu Dawud, Tirmidhi and Nasa'i have recorded that the Messenger of Allah (saws) said: "Anyone who recites Surah Al-Ikhlas and the mu'awwadhatain (i.e. Surah Al-Falaq and An-Nas) morning and evening, they shall be sufficient for him."

22. Make sure you get enough sleep during the night. If you are up for prayers, take naps during the day.

23. Be confident! Subhan'Allah, our bodies make metabolic adaptations to fasting, ensuring that milk production is not affected. In other words, our milk supply is inherently protected.

24. If you are feeling overwhelmed, let someone know. Take a break from fasting for a day or two.

25. If you feel like you are losing control of your emotions or are angry, pray taw'waz (authu billahi minash-shaitan ar-rajim), make wudu to "cool off" and/or lie down on the floor.

Chapter 11

Not Fasting? Stay Busy

Breastfeeding women who are not fasting often feel "left out" during Ramadan. However, Ramadan is not only about abstaining from food and drink. This time of self-purification and restraint is designed to help us attain taqwa so that we can be closer to our Creator. Therefore, there are many things a woman can do to engage in more acts of ibadah (worship), just like everyone else.

Here are some tips to help you feel included this Ramadan:

- Adhkar- Keep your tongue moist with the remembrance of Allah (swt).

- Cook and Serve Others- Prepare food for guests at your home or for the community iftar at your local masjid. If you know a family in need or who could use the help, cook in advance and deliver it to them before sundown. If you can't cook, buy dates, drinks, sweets, bread or fruit to give to others.

- Dua- Make dua as much as you like. Remember, dua is the essence of worship!

- Quran- If you are not in state where you can't touch the Quran, make it a priority to recite and memorize Quran each day. You can also benefit by listening to recitation more often during the day.

- Sadaqa- Give money towards charity.

- Tawbah & Istigfar- Repent and ask Allah (swt) for forgiveness of your sins.

- Community Service Participate in activities that involve helping others or the environment.

- Salat- Pray fard prayers on time. Focus on developing your khushu. If you wish, make extra prayers.

- Sunnah- Make more of an effort to practice the sunnah with everything you do.

- Salawat- Send blessings upon the Prophet Muhammad (saws).

- Reflection- Ponder about death and the Day of Judgment.

- Jumuah- Listen to the khutbah attentively and think about its message.

- Protect your Spiritual State- Make more of an effort to guard your eyes, ears and tongue from harmful interference.

- Take care of your body by eating tayyib, halal foods.

- Keep yourself clean and groomed.

- Set an alarm to wake up each night to worship Allah (swt).

- Attend or host qiyams for women.

Chapter 12

Make-Up Fasts

Every good action is rewarded by ten times its kind, up to seven hundred times, except fasting, which is for Me, and I reward it.-Tirmidhi, Muwatta

For each fast you miss, make up one day of fasting. Pregnant and nursing women are required to make up their fasts, if they are capable. Alternate days can be randomly chosen in the following months or years. But, it is better to make them up with diligence.

The month of Ramadhan [is that] in which was revealed the Qur'an, a guidance for the people and clear proofs of guidance and criterion. So whoever sights [the new moon of] the month, let him fast it; and whoever is ill or on a journey - then an equal number of other days. Allah intends for you ease and does not intend for you hardship and [wants] for you to complete the period and to glorify Allah for that [to] which He has guided you; and perhaps you will be grateful. Al Baqarah, Verse 185

Oh No! I Didn't Make-up My Missed Fasts from Last Year!

I recently stumbled upon an online debate among sisters about whether or not a breastfeeding mother had to make-up her missed fasts from Ramadan. Despite the fact that Allah (swt) has been merciful by given the breastfeeding woman a dispensation to be excused from fasting during the holy month, many of the women in the group felt that it was too much of a hardship to make-up those missed fasts. As a mother of four children born very close together, I know that it can be challenging to make-up fasts. However, whether we are still breastfeeding, pregnant with the next child, or have some other excuse for delaying, it is still obligatory to compensate for those fasts and Allah (swt) is the final judge. Islam is designed to make ease for us, and insh'Allah we can do better at fulfilling the debts we owe to Allah (swt).

Making of Missed Fasts

It is obligatory to make up missed fasts. No expiation is required for delaying. They can be made up gradually. Mothers should make up fasts as soon as possible to clear their debt with Allah. However, it does not have to be immediate. "And whosoever of you is sick or on a journey, (then fast the same) number of other days" (Surah Al Baqarah, Verse 185). However, one should be careful because if one dies without having taken reasonable means to make up the fasts without an excuse for delaying, then one would be considered sinful. One should keep track of unmade-up fasts. In case one dies unexpectedly, arrangements should be made for expiation payments to be given from the discretionary third of one's wealth upon death.

Feed the Poor

The breastfeeding woman is compared to someone with continuous hardship in fasting. She may not fast for one year during pregnancy, and 1-2 years of breastfeeding. That's almost 3 years. If you are too sick to make-up fasts anytime in the future, have back-to-back pregnancies or are nursing for several continuous years, you have the option to feed a poor person two meals for thirty days or pay the equivalent sadaqah of sixty meals. Fidya is an amount of money or food that is paid to the poor by the one who is not likely to be able to make up fasts due to great hardship. It also applies to those who have long lasting medical conditions that make them unable to fast currently and in the future. **If you are capable of fasting after nursing, even if another Ramadan passes, or your condition is expected to improve, plan to make-up your fasts by actually fasting.**

Action Plan

Make a chart to track your missed fasts. Check them off as you finish. After the days of Eid, if possible, make up 2-3 days a week in Shawwal. The momentum from Ramadan will make it much easier.

It is also wise to wait until winter when the days are shorter. Form a club of sisters online or in person that will make up fasts each month and encourage each other.

Year	Completed Fasts	Missed Fasts	Reason	Done?

1. Each month, mark the days you plan to fast on a calendar. Fast a few days each week.

2. Plan to fast on the White Days, the 13th, 14th, and 15th on a

lunar calendar. An Islamic calendar will match the corresponding days on the Gregorian calendar.

3. Mondays and Thursdays are sunnah days.

4. Write down all the duas you want to make while fasting.

Chapter 13

Food Journal

Write what you eat and how much you drink everyday. Include notes on how you feel, goals and any changes with your child.

Day 1

Day 2

Day 3

Day 4

Day 5

Day 6

Day 7

Day 8

Day 9

Day 10

Day 11

Day 12

Day 13

Day 14

Day 15

Day 16

Day 17

Day 18

Day 19

Day 20

Day 21

Day 22

Day 23

Day 24

Day 25

Day 26

Day 27

Day 28

Day 29

Day 30

Chapter 14

Eid Mubarak

Alhamdulilah, you made it through another Ramadan. Enjoy the celebrations and be sure to give yourself a treat. If your supply dipped, it will take time to return to normal. If you started supplementing, it may need to be continued until your supply is back up.

Chapter 15

Bibliography

Alyoumen, AlMasry (August, 2010) Five secrets for staying hydrated during Ramadan Ahmed Ramadan Published in Almasry Alyoum www.masress.com/en/almasryalyoumen/73186
–Sahih Muslim.
Ansari, Ustadha Zaynab, Badrudduja, Ustadha Sulma (2009) Pregnant Women and Fasting. URL:www.seekershub.com
Association, Australian breastfeeding , (August, 2014) Religious fasting and breastfeeding.www.breastfeeding.asn.au/bfinfo/religious-fasting-and-breastfeeding
Bajaj, Sarita, Khan, Afreen (2013) Women's Health in Ramadan by Chapter 75, pdf online. apiindia.org/medicine_update_2013/chap75.pdf
Begum, Lotifa (June, 2014) Avoiding Burnout in Ramadan. http://productivemuslim.com/avoid-burnout-during-ramadan/
Bheekoo-Shah, Fatima (June, 2014) Will you continue breastfeeding while fasting. URL: www.onsialm.net
Bonyata, Kelly (2012) Breastfeeding and Religious Fasting. kellymom.com/nutrition/mothers-diet/fasting/
Dawoud, Karimah Bint (June, 2014) Ready, Set, Go! Food & Nutrition for a Healthy Ramadan. muslimmatters.org/2014/06/22/ramadan-ready-set-go/

Hamza, Feras (2013) Tafsir al-Jalalayn Translation, Royal Aal al-Bayt Institute for Islamic Thought, Amman, Jordan

Hussein, Asmaa (June, 2015) Worship Smart, Not Hard www.ruqayasbookshelf.com

International, Sahih (January, 2016) Multiple quran verse translations. www.quran.com

Islam Community Page, Facebook (2012 What exactly is Rizq? www.facebook.com/ShareIslam/posts/350635591642011

Il'Adi, Anver (1999) Infants, Parents and Wet Nurses: Medieval Islamic Views on Breastfeeding and Their Social Implications. Brill

Jannah, Destination January, 2014) Halimah's Blessing. Episode 12: Seerah Life of the Prophets. www.destinationjannah.tumblr.com.

Khan, Zeba (2013) What I learned from not fasting. muslimmatter.com

Mendes, Carly (January, 2014) Nourishing Bone Broth. www.carleymendes.com

NHS Choices (2012). Ramadan health FAQs. http://www.nhs.uk/livewell/healthyramadan/pages/faqs.aspxAccessed30/7/13

Neville MC, Sawicki VS, Hay WW Jr (1993), Effects of fasting, elevated plasma glucose and plasma insulin concentrations on milk secretion in women. J Endocrinol 139(1):165–73.

Picciano, Mary Francis (2010). Comparative Lactation, Humans, University of Illinois Urbana-Champaign. ansci.illinois.edu/static/ansc438/Lactation/humans.html

Me, MumLoves (2012) Alternatives when you can't fast. www.mumlovesme.com

Mirza, Dr. Naomi (June, 2014) Breastfeeding in Ramadan. www.thedailystar.net/breastfeeding-during-ramadan-29813

Leiper, J.B.; Molla, A.M. (2003) Effects on health of fluid restriction during fasting in Ramadan. European Journal of Clinical Nutrition 57, Suppl 2, S30–S38

Rabbani, Faraz (2013) Breastfeeding and Fasting, Answers. www.seekershub.com

Rakicioğlu N, Samur G, Topçu A, Topçu AA (2006), The effect of

Ramadan on maternal nutrition and composition of breast milk. Pediatr Int 48(3):278–83.

Riodan, Jan (2005) Breastfeeding and Human Lactation. Bartlett.

Stacey Greaves-Favors, (2014) Pregnancy, Nursing and Ramadan `muslimink.com`

Smith, Anne (2015) Increasing Milk Supply. `www.breastfeedingbasics.com`

Tigas S, Sunehag A, Haymond MW (2002), Metabolic adaptation to feeding and fasting during lactation in humans. J Clin Endocrinol Metab 87(1):302–7.

Umm, Maryam (September, 2009) Ramadan Fasting for pregnant and lactating mothers. `www.islamisperfect.wordpress.com`

Wehr, Hans, and J. Milton. Cowan (1976) A Dictionary of Modern Written Arabic: (Arabic-English). N.p.: n.p., n.d. Print.

WellnessMama, Katie (2015) Herbal Nursing Mom Tea. `www.wellnessmama.com`

Zimmerman DR, Goldstein L, Lahat E, Braunstein R, Stahi D, Bar-Haim A, Berkovitch M (2009), Effect of a 24+ hour fast on breast milk composition. J Hum Lact 25(2):194–8.